Praise for *Be Your Own Shaman*

*"Deborah King's newest book, **Be Your Own Shaman**, is wisdom-filled, practical, and packed with information! Writing in a conversational style that's easy to read, Deborah leads us on an inner pilgrimage that shatters age-old misconceptions of energy healing. In doing so, she reminds us that we're born with nature's most powerful instrument of healing—the gift to be able to sense and direct subtle energy through our bodies. In addition to demonstrating our ability to heal, this book instills within us the confidence to experience the benefit of such a force in our own lives. Whether you're a novice or an expert in the power of subtle energy, **Be Your Own Shaman** is a must-have for every library, and should be required reading for everyone with a passion for miracles."*

— **Gregg Braden**, the *New York Times* best-selling
author of *The Divine Matrix* and *Fractal Time*

"This book is an essential guide for all seekers of higher truth who are destined to fulfill their purpose of helping others by first healing themselves."

— **Neale Donald Walsch**, the *New York Times* best-selling
author of *Conversations with God* and *The Mother of Invention*

"Deborah King is a courageous and gifted healer."

— **Christiane Northrup, M.D.**, the *New York Times* best-selling author of
Women's Bodies, Women's Wisdom and *The Secret Pleasures of Menopause*

"Happiness comes by living our true nature. Deborah King's book opens us up to realizing the powerful healing nature that lives within us all."

— **Robert Holden, Ph.D.**, the best-selling
author of *Be Happy* and *Happiness Now!*

"I love the mix of esoteric and practical wisdom, the confluence of ancient and modern healing traditions!"

— **Marci Shimoff**, the *New York Times*
best-selling author of *Happy for No Reason*

"Along with at least 50 other seekers, sufferers, and spectators, I'm here to witness one of King's . . . Truth Healings, a free event at which she offers to treat anyone who will publicly put himself in her healing hands. . . . King's demonstration has been electrifying. . . . The next day I call her office to book a private appointment, which will prove to be the strangest, most exciting hour I've had in my yearlong experiment in alternative medicine, Hollywood style."

— **Kevin West**, editor of *W* magazine, from "Healing, Hollywood Style"

BE
YOUR
OWN
SHAMAN

ALSO BY DEBORAH KING

Truth Heals: What You Hide <u>Can</u> Hurt You*

Truth Heals Cards

Truth Heals Journal

*Available from Hay House

Hay House USA: www.hayhouse.com®
Hay House Australia: www.hayhouse.com.au
Hay House UK: www.hayhouse.co.uk
Hay House South Africa: www.hayhouse.co.za
Hay House India: www.hayhouse.co.in

❖ ❖

BE YOUR OWN SHAMAN

HEAL YOURSELF AND OTHERS WITH 21ST-CENTURY ENERGY MEDICINE

DEBORAH KING

HAY HOUSE, INC.
Carlsbad, California • New York City
London • Sydney • Johannesburg
Vancouver • Hong Kong • New Delhi

Published and distributed in the United States by: Hay House, Inc.: www
.hayhouse.com • *Published and distributed in Australia by:* Hay House
Australia Pty. Ltd.: www.hayhouse.com.au • *Published and distributed in the
United Kingdom by:* Hay House UK, Ltd.: www.hayhouse.co.uk • *Published and
distributed in the Republic of South Africa by:* Hay House SA (Pty), Ltd.: www
.hayhouse.co.za • *Distributed in Canada by:* Raincoast: www.raincoast.com •
Published in India by: Hay House Publishers India: www.hayhouse.co.in

Editorial supervision: Jill Kramer • *Project editor:* Patrick Gabrysiak
Indexer: Richard Comfort: rcomfort8608@att.net • *Design:* Tricia Breidenthal

Library of Congress Cataloging-in-Publication Data

King, Deborah
  Be your own shaman : heal yourself and others with 21st-century energy medi-
cine / Deborah King.
      p. cm.
  Includes index.
  ISBN 978-1-4019-3078-3 (hardcover : alk. paper) 1. Healing. 2. Shamanism. I.
Title.
  RZ400.K547 2011
  615.5--dc22
                              2010034788

Tradepaper ISBN: 978-1-4019-3079-0
Digital ISBN: 978-1-4019-3080-6

15 14 13 12   7 6 5 4
1st edition, March 2011
4th edition, March 2012

Printed in the United States of America

*I dedicate this book to all
those who have sought my help over
the years, in my teaching programs, in my
workshops, and at speaking engagements.
Your belief that it is possible to live your
lives fully—despite the past—and your
faith, give this book its spirit.*

CONTENTS

INTRODUCTION

Sometime ago, at a conference where I was speaking and doing healing work with audience volunteers, a woman named Anna joined me onstage. She told me that she was 49 years old, had severe hypertension, and didn't do well with the medications her doctors had tried with her. Her blood pressure remained dangerously high, and she and her doctors were worried that she might suffer a sudden stroke. Anna had been following their orders to the letter—watching her diet and getting plenty of regular exercise —but still, her blood pressure remained too high. Fearing for her life, and desperate to know what else she could do, Anna had come to the conference for help.

After hearing her story, I began my work by "feeling" into Anna's human energy field—that's the field of energy that both surrounds and penetrates the body. There, I found emotions from her childhood that she had never fully processed: anger, fear, and self-hatred that had developed at the age of 12 when her mother and father had gotten divorced. As children so often do, Anna had blamed herself for her parents' unhappiness and breakup. During my assessment, I discerned that it was these unprocessed emotions that had formed an energetic block in her cardiovascular system, and that they were the underlying cause of her blood-pressure condition.

In the space of just a few minutes, using a method I developed after decades of studying and working with healers around the world, I cleared those old, destructive emotions from Anna's field and physical self. I then gave her a hug and sent her on her way, knowing that with the blockage in her energy field now removed, her body could heal itself.

Anna contacted me a few months later, saying that her blood pressure had dramatically improved. Not only was she no longer at risk of having an imminent stroke, but her doctors had reduced her medication. She thanked me profusely for helping her get her life back.

How did I produce this shift in Anna's health so quickly? Well . . . by using ancient techniques that you, too, can learn to help heal yourself as well as others.

Our Human History

Thousands of years ago, we knew how to heal others the way that I helped Anna. We lived in tribes, close to our mother, the earth. We were intimately connected to one another and to our Source. We communicated telepathically, and could talk to our deceased ancestors. We could talk to the animals, too.

Every one of us had a special talent—an innate gift that was ours to develop and pursue, blessing our communities with the fruits of our labors. Some of us excelled at music or were adept with herbs. Some were leaders. Some of us had the special talent of levitating, walking through walls, or bilocating (being in two places at once). Or perhaps we could predict the future. But if our special gift was the ability to heal—to attract, transmit, and direct healing energy—we were given the title of *shaman*.

Over time, as our world became more analytical, we relied less on our special gifts and, sadly, began to lose them. Most human beings today possess only remnants of what once was. We may have, for example, gotten a glimpse from time to time of these talents in our own lives—a *knowing* about who's on the phone before it rings, the *sense* that our child is hurt before we get the call, or that sinking *feeling* that our partner is cheating on us before he or she confesses. These are the last vestiges of the abilities we all enjoyed millennia ago. They provided us with valuable information and skills that allowed our communities to flourish and empowered us to thrive as individuals.

The good news is that the template for these gifts still resides within us—in the memory of our cells, as part of our DNA. With a little awareness, attention, and practice, those ancient gifts can be reclaimed and put back into use, including the healing power of the shaman.

Shaman, Healer, and Co-creator

So what does it mean to be a shaman today? Is it someone who wears a feathered headdress, shakes a rattle, and dances around a fire to the beating of drums as he communes with an invisible world of spirits? It could be. But did you know that the sweet little old church lady with blue hair and clothes from the 1950s could be a shaman, too?

I use the word *shaman* to mean "a healer"—someone who expands his or her consciousness and conducts healing energy to help others resolve whatever is ailing them on the physical, mental, emotional, and spiritual planes. Most of all, shamans are people from any background who have done the requisite work to heal *themselves*—clearing away blocked and stagnant energy, releasing past traumas, connecting with guides in the spiritual realms, and listening deep within so that they are aligned to fulfill their potential and pursue their highest life purpose.

Just like every other human, *you can be your own shaman*. The gift of healing ourselves is not limited to the select few who have the potential to treat others. Rather, every one of us is a natural-born self-healer—these abilities are there within us, even if they've been dormant. Our task, then, is to learn how to access and use them. To do that, we must familiarize ourselves with, and begin to explore, the hidden world of healing energy that resides within and all around us. Helping you do that is my purpose in writing this book.

One reason why I use the term *shaman,* which can also be defined as a person who acts as an intermediary between the human world and spirit worlds—between the natural and supernatural—is that it encapsulates the idea that everything in our universe is connected. We are all linked—to each other, to the physical world of our senses, and to the world beyond that we aren't able to see. *We are all one,* much more so than most of us realize. Outside of our individual identities and boundaries within this tangible reality, we live in one massive energy soup, connected to everything else. Quantum physics is in the process of proving exactly that. And it is in this infinite place of Oneness that healing originates and occurs. Our goal, then, for those of us who want to heal, is to reside in this space.

Any number of different paths can lead us there. Contemporary 21st-century healers stand on the shoulders of all the sages and shamans who have come before them—from ancient times, beginning thousands of years ago, to the modern era—spanning a vast array of religious and cultural affiliations. Every culture on Earth has had some form of shamanic practice, and at the heart of every one of those traditions is a path that leads us back to Source, the universal energy that is the Creator of All That Is.

In fact, healing is a co-creative process—it always requires a partnership between you and Source. No shaman or medical doctor, healer or therapist, herbal remedy or manufactured drug can heal you on its own. For healing to occur, there must always be a part of you, even if it's completely unconscious, that elects to participate. It's the part that freely chooses to be a force in your own transformation. Nevertheless, the more clarity, balance, and openness you bring to healing, the more easily you will be able to receive that outpouring of grace.

Introduction

You may not feel that you have been adequately prepared for shamanhood, but that's not true. To illustrate how your life so far may have put you on this path, I'll share a bit of my own story.

How I Became a Shaman (and You Can, Too)

If you have read my first book, *Truth Heals: What You Hide Can Hurt You;* have seen me on TV; or have heard me speak in person or on my weekly Hay House Radio show, you may already know a little about my background. If not, allow me to share it with you now.

I survived a pretty horrendous childhood, filled with sexual and emotional abuse. My mother despised and resented me, and did all she could to diminish me and control my every move. Her parenting was downright cruel. My father, on the other hand, absolutely adored me, but mixed his affection with a compulsion to repeat his own sexually abusive childhood. He molested me from the time I was a toddler until the age of 12, and raped me for the first time at age 9. Our local parish priest, to whom my father confessed his abhorrent behavior, also sexually abused me at the same age. My mother always turned a blind eye.

From a young age, the actions of both my parents caused me to become hypervigilant. I'm sure I had post-traumatic stress disorder by the time I was four. Abused children are always waiting for the other shoe to drop—the footsteps that mean the abuser is heading their way—so they get very sensitive to even miniscule changes in their environment. As is common with these kids, the trauma of my childhood put my tender young nervous system on such high alert that I instinctively developed the ability to go into a heightened state of awareness in an effort to stay safe. In this condition, I could see, hear, feel, and know beyond what we think of as "ordinary." Thus began my training as a shaman.

Expanding My Awareness

As it turns out, my traumatic childhood was teeming with opportunities to expand my own awareness and develop an ever-deepening connection with Source. As a child, I learned to read not only between the lines of what was being said, but also between the glances, gestures, and emotional nuances of that which was too painful to see, let alone articulate. I began to read deeply into others . . . to sense their hidden motives, deepest fears, and darkest demons. It was a resourceful way to survive an unpredictable, and often treacherous, environment. Long before I stepped foot in a courtroom to do battle in my first career as an attorney, I had become a skilled negotiator with the dark side of people and life.

As a small child, I also stayed very connected to Source—that force many call "Spirit," "God," or whatever term works best for you. Because young children have recently come from Source—it's where they were just prior to their birth—it's relatively easy for them to head back there if they get frightened. Their consciousness simply escapes right out of their bodies.

Between the ages of 6 and 14, I spent hours and hours on my knees, praying in front of pictures and statues. Ironically, I was asking mostly for forgiveness for what I assumed were my sins. Like all children, I blamed myself for my family's problems. Having been raised Catholic, I found it easy to connect to iconic figures such as Jesus, Mary, and all of the saints. Had I been brought up in another tradition, it would have been *its* enlightened masters that I would have been praying to.

Another one of my survival techniques as a child was to spend as much time as possible outside. Every day after school, and after practicing the piano and finishing my homework, I would go outdoors to get away from my oppressive home life. I loved to sit in nature and simply *be*. I remember spending at least an hour every evening and all weekend communing with the trees, the rocks, and the animals. I felt very safe there. This was another easy way for me to shift into expanded awareness.

My spiritual experiences, combined with the trauma of my abuse and tendency to spend time in nature, taught me how to enter into a heightened state—the same level of consciousness that is required to attract, conduct, and transmit universal energy for healing. In addition, without even knowing it, I was perfecting my ability to connect to spiritual beings—ancestors, angels, and saints—who are instrumental in effecting healing.

My Big Wake-Up Call

Everything changed when I hit puberty, as it so often does. I rejected all that I knew and everything I had learned. When I rebelled against my family, I was promptly sent away to boarding school, where I stopped going into expanded states and quit using my extrasensory abilities. I completely divorced myself from my spiritual connection, replacing it with alcohol and prescription drugs, cigarettes and promiscuity—whatever altered my consciousness so I wouldn't feel a thing. I had no idea that I was totally out of touch with my body and my feelings.

I became anxious and depressed. I took terrible care of myself and seldom ate. Obsessed with wearing a size 2, I was always on one extreme diet or another and smoked excessively to control my weight. Even though I looked great on the outside, I was a real mess on the inside. Yet somehow I made it through high school, college, and law school, and started my career as an attorney. I'd only worked a year when, at age 25, I was told the words no one ever wants to hear: *You have cancer.* After a decade of numbing and running, my roadway had run out. Being diagnosed with cancer was a *major* wake-up call.

I immediately decided that I didn't want the radical surgery that was the treatment for cervical cancer at the time; I was young and didn't want any of my reproductive organs removed. So I kept postponing the surgery while searching for other options. I also spent a great deal of time thinking about what might have *caused* my cancer. I suspected that there was an emotional component, but I was so far removed from who I was that I couldn't name even a single emotion I had . . . except for fear. I knew that I was afraid of the surgery, afraid of losing my organs, and afraid of dying. With a deep belief that true healing comes from within and a tremendous desire to heal, I set out to see if I could find the answer to getting well for myself.

My healing journey started with Alcoholics Anonymous, where I quit both alcohol and prescription drugs the very first day. Being free of substances was the first step in gaining the clarity I needed to get to the bottom of my cancer—to figuring out its cause as well as how to recover from it. Interestingly, I found that all 12-step programs offer an opportunity to reconnect with Source, and I was quickly able to reforge the spiritual connection I had abandoned as a teen.

At the same time, I developed a daily practice of meditation, which is the single greatest thing I've ever done for myself. Meditation puts us in the present, completely relaxes the body and mind, and takes away stress—not to mention that it makes us look and feel younger! Most important for me, though, was that it reconnected me to Source and gave me more of that lucidity I needed to address my disease.

Feeling good about my new choices, I decided to continue my quest for alternatives to surgery. I became acquainted with acupuncture. I then tried massage to get in touch with my body, and I took up journaling to rediscover my emotions. Everywhere I went, I carried a little notebook in which I would jot down whatever I was feeling, as often as every half hour. I wrote it all in that little notebook, pouring my heart out—how I really felt about my childhood and my family; how inadequate I felt in my job; and, of course, how envious I was of all the women out there who I was sure were thinner and prettier than I was. As I did so, I discovered that giving my emotions expression through writing without judging them was a huge step in becoming aware of what was going on inside of me.

I also tried a treatment called *energy healing* in a series of sessions with a healer. That's when, the next thing I knew, I had a total remission from the cancer.

How I Healed

I realized that my drastic improvement had resulted from the combination of meditating, keeping track of my emotions through journaling, and the energy work. These practices had helped me become aware of, and process out, the toxic emotions I'd been harboring. Deep down, I *knew* that it was the feelings I had never dealt with from my abusive childhood that had made me so sick, and that it was moving those emotions out of my body and mind that had laid the foundation for getting well.

Intrigued by my clean bill of health, I wanted to understand how it had happened and be able to reproduce it for others who were ill. Even more, I wanted to show them how to avoid getting sick in the first place.

I began to study healing with an esoteric Christian group who had mastered "distance healing," which they called "prayer," and I spent the next ten years working with them. I also enrolled in an advanced meditation course, which led me to the study of the ancient Vedas—the oldest scriptures of the East Indians. Later, I attended a *Mystery School*—a place for studying metaphysical mysteries, the purpose of which is to forge a connection with our deeper spirit, and thus with all of life. The program I attended focused on the human energy field and chakra system, also derived from early Vedic knowledge, and it was there that I first learned what is commonly referred to as energy, or "hands-on," healing—the same form of treatment that had helped me heal from cancer. I spent many years in that field, working with individual clients and teaching energy work.

During those years, I kept my day job as an attorney so that I could devote every free moment and spare dollar to furthering my exploration of these concepts. At that time, there weren't many people in what was then acknowledged as a highly mystical field. My family and quite a few of my friends thought I was crazy to be jetting around the globe spending my time and money on apprenticeships with masters, shamans, and priests. And when I was home, my habit of getting up in the wee hours of the morning and driving to a nearby secluded monastery to meditate for hours on end was considered unusual at best.

Stepping into Shamanhood

Much to my disappointment, while I was always very intuitive and had a burning desire to learn, I didn't seem to have any special talent for effecting healings. In fact, many, many years of study and practice went by during which I was sure I was wasting my time because I'd accomplished so little in the way of actually curing others. Still, I never stopped trying and meditating, believing that *this* was the key to developing healing abilities.

Well, those formative years ended up proving invaluable, as they helped me get a handle on my ego—the nemesis of every healer. I needed to shed my overdeveloped lawyer's bravado, let go of my obsession with my appearance, and become humble enough to be the handmaiden of Spirit. Several of my apprenticeships with shamans were grueling and some even demeaning, which helped me cultivate that much-needed humility. During my time with one master healer, the other apprentices called me "Cinderella" because I was always given the least desirable, least prestigious job —as far back in the room and away from the action—as possible.

Then, after years of studying with various spiritual leaders and practicing their techniques, as well as spending countless hours in an intensive state of meditation and prayer, I developed a powerful healing method of my own: a combination of what I learned from various teachers, coupled with ancient techniques that I accessed directly from the unified field—the universal Source from which all information and healing comes. It was in using this new technique that real physical change started to occur literally right under my hands! I received what I had longed for and worked so hard toward: *the gift of healing.* Today, I travel the world teaching, demonstrating my work, and sharing this gift. But I never forget that, as a healer, I am only a facilitator in this miraculous co-creative process between the person being healed and Source.

Introduction

✤ ✤

On the surface, it may seem that my start in the corporate world was an aberration from my true path. But I soon realized that my career as an attorney, not to mention my abusive childhood, had been blessings in disguise. One of the tasks involved in effecting healing transformations in others is forming unbending intent—the same kind, ironically, that wins lawsuits. So much of the left-brained, linear, analytical thinking that I learned in law school and practiced as an attorney became surprisingly handy in this field of energy medicine.

So whatever your particular journey has been, rest assured that nothing happens in your life that isn't part of your Divine plan. Everything will serve your higher purpose in some way.

Take a moment now to re-imagine your own story, to see the obstacles and traumas and disciplines of your life as the necessary foundation for your development as a "wounded healer." Ask yourself what may have prepared you to develop this gift of being able to heal yourself and possibly others. Are you focused, sensitive, compassionate, hardworking? Do you frequently spend time in nature, meditation, or prayer? Have you begun to work through the wounds and emotional issues from your childhood? The list of possible experiences, qualities, and skills you already possess to help you in this endeavor is endless.

Real healing power *is* inside you; it just needs to be awakened, nurtured, and practiced. You *can* be your own shaman, and this book will start you on your way.

Within These Pages

In the following chapters, I present you with clues, pathways, and exercises that will help you engage with the world of spirit and bring you into harmony with the sacred energy of all of life. It is in this creative space that you will access the power to heal.

The book is organized into ten chapters that take you through a progression of what energy medicine is, how it works, and how you can begin expanding your consciousness to access its tremendous power. I'll take you on a quick journey back in time to discover the history of energy medicine throughout the ages, as well as the world's most accomplished and recognized healers. You will then examine your thoughts to eradicate those that may prevent you from being able to develop the skills of the shaman. With any limiting beliefs out of the way, you will then be ready to learn about and develop your shamanic gifts—the extrasensory perceptions that are the hallmark of this work.

Next, I'll teach you the five key practices that will help you continue your expansion and be an integral part of your development and effectiveness as a healer. You'll also journey to the dark side, looking at different forms of psychic attack as well as how you can protect yourself from them. At this point, you'll be ready to practice some healing techniques and learn about others that are amazing and jaw-dropping. The book concludes with some pitfalls to look out for and goals to aspire to as you walk the path of the shaman.

You'll find numerous exercises throughout the book—they have been included in certain sections where experiential practice will assist in your understanding of the concepts being presented. I highly recommend using a notebook or journal for the exercises that require writing, which can then be used for what I hope will be your new practice of daily journal writing. My goal is for you to take advantage of these methods for expanding your awareness, bringing you in touch with what lies within, and creating greater harmony.

After reading this book, you may very well find that your ability to sense what others are thinking and feeling has heightened, and that you have the ability to connect more easily to the spirit of your deceased love ones, just as your ancestors could. Your dreams will become more vivid and give you important information about your life, while you realize that nagging physical problems such as high blood pressure or issues with addiction or depression have diminished or disappeared. These will all be signs that you are reconnecting to your deepest Source—a vast, unlimited field of information and power where you can achieve anything you want, including self-healing.

Honoring Your Beliefs

It's also important for you to know that I will never infringe upon or violate any of your personal religious beliefs, whatever they may be. You may be Jewish or Christian or Muslim or Hindu or Buddhist or into the 12 steps or a believer in the forces of Nature; or, perhaps you have created your own spiritual belief system that incorporates elements from many different traditions, as I have. Whatever your beliefs, and I hope they are always evolving, I encourage you to deepen them and practice them with devotion.

You will find that your study of healing will inevitably lead you to a deeper spiritual connection, as it's impossible to expand your consciousness and increase your awareness without becoming more connected to Source. You will always know when something does or doesn't feel right for you, as healing is simply a natural extension of being in right relationship with yourself and the natural world.

Welcome to a stepping-stone on the path to becoming your own shaman. As the traditional Navajo prayer says, "May you walk in beauty in your partnership with the universe."

❖ ❖ ❖ ❖

chapter one

WHAT IS ENERGY MEDICINE?

I wrote this book for one simple reason: *I want you to know that you can experience healing.* You can learn how to heal yourself, and even help others heal.

It's true. Actual, bona fide healings happen right now in the 21st century. Cancer vanishes. Arthritis goes away. A lifetime filled with deep, dark, soul-crushing depression suddenly lifts. I have personally taken part in healings that were astonishingly dramatic. While these healings may seem miraculous, it's good to keep in mind that a miracle is simply something for which we don't yet have an explanation . . . but that isn't to say that one doesn't exist.

Medical doctors aren't comfortable with the word *miracles.* Instead, they refer to them as "spontaneous remissions" while shaking their collective heads in wonder. They think in terms of curing the symptoms of a disease through pharmaceuticals and surgeries, rather than going deeper to heal the condition that caused the affliction to begin with. Take diabetes, for example. Doctors will help you manage it, but they do not have a cure. Diabetes can, however, be cured with energy medicine. *All* disease can. In fact, its "miracles" are not limited to physical healing. Energy medicine can heal what ails us in every area of our lives.

I'm sure you have something you want to heal. We all do. Your health, your weight, your finances, a relationship—or even the lack of one. And maybe you not only want to heal the parts of your life that are dysfunctional, but you are also intrigued, as I was, by the idea of being able to help others. The fascinating thing is that these two goals, healing yourself and healing others, are inextricably linked: in the process of learning to facilitate healing in others, you yourself become healed. It's actually *impossible* for you to study energy medicine without experiencing positive change yourself.

Energy as Medicine

What is energy medicine? It's a dynamic process that merges, as the name implies, two very powerful things: *energy* and *medicine*. Even though we can't usually see it, energy is all around us, existing in a variety of wavelengths and frequencies. It includes cosmic radiation, x-rays, radio waves, infrared waves, and a more subtle form that permeates the entire universe and comprises everything within it, including you and me. This is the foundation of energy medicine, and what we'll be talking about here. This force, upon which our universe runs, is intelligent, alive, and the source of all life. In this infinite field of potential, creativity knows no bounds and anything is possible. Inexhaustible, it has no beginning and no end.

The ancients knew all about this conscious and creative energy: how it penetrates all space, flows from one object to another, and connects a thing to everything else. We call this field of all possibilities the *universal energy field,* or simply the *unified field.*

Ironically, what seers took for granted thousands of years ago, our present-day scientists are only beginning to understand. Today's researchers are on the brink of being able to use scientific instruments to record the unified field. It's likely that modern science will soon discover that the energy that constitutes the unified field is a much finer substance than anything previously known.

Until then, this magnificent force—invisible to most of the human race—will likely remain a mystery. However, with training and practice, it can be accessed. In fact, I've learned almost all of what I know about this field experientially—that is, while in prayer, in meditation, and conducting energy in the practice of healing. The unified field holds every fact and facet of the universe, from the beginning of time through the present and into the limitless future, along with the energy that can be harnessed to effect change, including that which happens at the cellular level of the human body.

For our purposes, then, energy medicine is the employment of this inexhaustible field as a factor to treat disease—that's what *medicine* means. In this Divine application, *energy is the medicine.* And in connecting to this universal field—attracting, conducting, and transmitting its energy to effect healing in yourself and others—you become the healer. *You become a shaman.*

While this kind of medicine in its various forms dates back to the dawn of human history, it is also as new as the most innovative medical technology in the most modern hospital on Earth. Energy medicine is completely natural; extremely safe; and, in my opinion, the most exciting new area available to study, perfect, and practice as a career. But above all, it is an incredibly powerful way to heal your own life.

The Shaman's Workspace: The Human Energy Field

As we saw with the example of Anna, whom you met in the first few pages of this book, one place where the shaman does his or her work is the *human energy field.* Also called the *aura,* it is a manifestation of the *universal energy field* that is the cornerstone of all life. My view of the human energy field in its expanded state started when I was quite young, during the time when I was engaging in conversation with pictures and statues of saints and representations of the Divine. All of these figures were depicted with halos of light circling their heads. When I later studied Eastern philosophy and religion as an adult, I found that saints from these traditions are also portrayed with a light surrounding their heads. Both representations show the human energy field in its more conscious form. Today, this same light can be seen by clairvoyants around the heads of those who are spiritually advanced.

The human energy field surrounds the entire body in what appear to be levels. Unlike the layers of an onion, though, these levels interpenetrate the body as well as each other, ultimately extending outward several feet or more beyond the skin. In most systems of thought, there are seven main levels, as well as numerous minor ones. Additionally, there are even more above the head. Each ascending level of the field is higher in frequency and vibration than the one below it. To use music as a metaphor, each one is similar to a higher octave.

The human energy field precedes the existence of the human body. In fact, your body arises directly out of your energy field. One analogy that's frequently used to illustrate this phenomenon is the phantom limb effect. People who lose a limb can often still feel it, as if it still exists. That's because it *does* still exist—on the level from which it originally came.

You can think of the human energy field as a living template for the body, which, consequently, ultimately mirrors what's happening in the field. Thus, any distortion or imbalance in your field will sooner or later negatively impact you physically. Likewise, if you make a correction in the field, a corresponding change will manifest in the body. It's imperative to understand that the levels of your field are not only as real as your physical self, but they are also, in some ways, even more consequential. This is why healing the field—restructuring it, rebalancing it, and charging it—is so important.

Like the unified field from which it comes, the human energy field is intelligent and alive. Because this is the realm in which your psychological processes take place, it's constantly changing in response to your consciousness. Its different levels correspond to different aspects of your life, and your experiences and emotional reactions will determine your field's state. This, in turn, affects the health of your body. If you consider that, you'll conclude, as I have, that all of life's problems, including physical disease, are psychosomatic—meaning they're created by thoughts and emotions. Just bear in mind, though, that the field itself doesn't *create* an event—it's the vehicle through which your consciousness affects your body as well as other areas of your life.

If one or more of your levels is weak, your life experiences that correspond to that same level may be equally weak. If it remains out of sync for a long time, you may very well develop health problems in the related physical area. Those who are intuitive can sense an illness in someone's energy field long before it shows up in his or her body. Thus, ailments or diseases can often be avoided by making the necessary "adjustments" in the energy field before they manifest. These adjustments are central to the work of energy medicine.

Energy Centers in the Human Body: The Chakras

In addition to levels, the human energy field is also organized into energy centers called *chakras*. A vast amount has been written on the chakras and their incredible influence on our lives, so I'll be including only a cursory overview of them here.

Chakra means "wheel of light" in Sanskrit, and each one looks a bit like a funnel or vortex that spins when it is operating optimally. As the chakras spin, there is a constant exchange of energy with the environment—going from them out into the world and from the unified field coming in. That incoming energy nurtures and supports our individual fields and physical bodies.

Like the levels of your own field, these centers of spinning energy correspond to, and heavily influence, different aspects of your life. For example, if your fourth chakra, the heart chakra, is dysfunctional, you won't be able to give or receive love and might have high blood pressure; and if your fifth chakra, the throat chakra, is not operational, you'll have a hard time finalizing creative projects and may have hypothyroidism. Therefore, it's crucial to both your emotional and physical health that the chakras are functioning properly.

And, like the levels of your field, the chakras are affected by your consciousness. If you get emotionally upset about something, these energy centers can become distorted or imbalanced; they may get lopsided or start spinning the wrong way. When that happens, they can cease bringing in new energy and only send it out, leaving your field depleted and making you susceptible to physical problems. Ideally, you want your chakras spinning gently and consistently in an energy exchange, and to be similar in shape and size to one another.

There are 7 major chakras and more than 20 minor ones corresponding to the body. Usually, we focus on the seven main ones, which start at the base of the spine and run to the top of the head. On the physical level, each of these is located close to a major nerve ganglion that comes out from your spinal column. The chakras are connected to your *vertical power current,* which you can think of as an energetic spine—the distinction being that this current actually widens and allows more energy to flow through it as you move up in consciousness and service to others.

Each chakra represents an aspect of consciousness that is essential to your life. As a system, they integrate your mind, body, and spirit; and each has a physical, emotional, creative, and celestial component. As your chakras open up more, you develop a deeper awareness of the state of that particular level. Perhaps you have one chakra that's a lot more open than others—for example, your heart chakra. Consequently, you will have more awareness of yourself and others in the "love and compassion" department.

Additionally, each chakra has its own purpose relative to the area of consciousness that it influences, which tends to make you lean a particular way or head in a certain direction. It's almost as though the chakra develops a mind of its own. For instance, someone who is very compassionate, like the Dalai Lama, will operate almost exclusively from his heart chakra. Actress Pamela Anderson, on the other hand, is fixated on her second chakra, the sexual energy center. For her, life is all about sensuality, and she is operating almost entirely from that area.

When Chakras Become Distorted

When we close our chakras or they spin the wrong way, we send our own energy out into the world. This is what a psychologist would call a *projection*. What we're doing is creating a reality that we believe to be valid, but in actuality is something that we fabricated from our childhood experiences.

For example, if a child's father abandons the family, the son may react by instinctively stopping the flow of love from himself to his father, thus blocking off and closing his heart chakra to protect himself from the pain of abandonment. Since our chakras not only metabolize energy but also sense it around us, this child will most likely perceive a state of non-love. He'll believe that the world is an unloving place and have no idea that he is sending out his own feelings. This is how we create our own psychological reality. Of course, if this child's fourth chakra remains closed throughout his life, that will affect his physical heart and related functions, like blood pressure and circulation.

This process works the same for every chakra. Whenever you block an experience you are having because it is unpleasant or frightening or hurtful, you also block the corresponding positive emotion that you would normally be sending out and receiving in that same chakra, which will ultimately cause it to become disfigured. It may get clogged with stagnant energy and spin irregularly or in the wrong direction, eventually becoming severely distorted or torn—the signs of a dysfunction manifesting. By the way, most people have at least a couple of chakras spinning the wrong way unless they've done a tremendous amount of personal work, meditation, and the like, so don't panic if you think yours aren't perfect. This book will help you right them.

While every human being and each chakra's activities are unique, there are sometimes common patterns. For example, it's rare for someone with fibromyalgia to have a correctly functioning first chakra. I've found that fibromyalgia patients are invariably dealing with a great deal of unexpressed fear, which shuts down their first chakra and inclines the body to pull away from the earth.

When this happens, they don't feel safe. Thus, those with this disorder inadvertently create the very situation they fear the most. (To learn more about the connection of the chakras to physical health, please see my book *Truth Heals: What You Hide Can Hurt You,* which is one of many resources that cover this topic in detail.) Contrast that to a well-functioning first chakra, which will spin properly and bring to the individual a world that feels safe.

EXERCISE: Chakra Meditation

To become acquainted with your own chakras, and to help restore them to a healthy flow, here's a basic meditation that you can do whenever you want to tune in to them—which also tunes them up! With practice, you will begin sensing the present state of each chakra—its relative health—and may even pick up other information about yourself as you explore. Note that you may want to read through this meditation before trying it.

Let's get started:

— Be seated comfortably and close your eyes. Take a deep breath. Let all the cares of the day fade away; let everything go. Take another deep breath and feel your feet on the floor. Feel your calves and knees, and then feel your thighs and buttocks on the chair.

— Breathe deeply and bring your attention to your first chakra, also called the *root* or *base* chakra, located at the base of your genitals. Bright red in color, this chakra is the seat of your physical existence and the foundation of your physical health. Intend for this chakra to be circling properly and gently, bringing energy from the earth, through your feet, up your legs, and right into that base chakra.

— Take another deep breath and move to the second chakra, known as the *sacral* or *sexual* chakra, located midway between your first chakra and your waistline. Its color is a vibrant orange. This is the seat of your emotional body, the center of all your connections to others. Picture it circling gently and expanding. Take another deep breath into this area.

— Now, while taking another deep breath, move to the third chakra, known as the *solar plexus* chakra. It is situated halfway between your navel and your breastbone. A beautiful bright yellow, this is your power center and the seat of your mental body, the place where you identify with your ego and self-esteem. Intend for it to be gently circling and expanding.

— Move up to the fourth, or *heart*, chakra, right in the center of your chest. Its color is a lovely kelly green. Breathe deeply into that area and feel it expand. This is the seat of your astral body, where the energy field connects to the astral plane (the bridge between the physical and spiritual levels of your energy field). It is the place where you connect with compassion, love, understanding, and care. Set an intention to express these characteristics. If you're like most people, you don't spend enough time truly appreciating yourself. Acknowledge your uniqueness, inner beauty, courage, and valor—all of the finest qualities of your highest self. Some of these features may not yet have been developed, but they're there. By focusing on the fourth chakra and intending, you're opening yourself to manifesting them in your life today.

— Take another breath and move up slightly to the thymus, which is located in the upper chest under your breastbone and just below your thyroid gland. Intend to have your thymus, which is the seat of immune functioning as well as spiritual development, expand. Breathe deeply into it and intend for it to be vibrant and healthy. Healing always begins with intention. Always.

— Breathe deeply and move up slightly to the cobalt blue fifth chakra, also called the *throat* chakra, right in the center of your throat. This is the seat of the blueprint for your physical body. Visualize and intend for it to be circling ever so gently, bringing new energy in, sending old energy out. Intend for your throat chakra to be open. See yourself singing, journaling, and expressing yourself in artistic, creative ways.

— Move up to the sixth chakra, also known as the *third eye* chakra, located in the center of your forehead, right between your eyebrows. Its color is violet, and it is the seat of the celestial body and the key to discernment. Take a breath and picture it circling and cycling ever so gently, bringing information to you and exposing you to other planes. Intend for it to open more widely so that you can see, intuit, and sense beyond this level.

— Move on to the seventh, or *crown*, chakra, right at the very top of your head with its radiant gold and white light. This is the seat of your connection to spirit, of prayer and meditation, spirituality, devotion, faith, and inspiration. Breathe, and intend for it to be open, circling gently and bringing energy to you from the universal field, from All That Is.

— And now move one higher to the eighth chakra, also called the *soul star*, located between one and three feet above your head. This is the seat of your higher self. Intend for it to open so that you can access and manifest your greatest qualities.

— Now take a deep breath and move your attention back to your body, back to your feet, back to the ground, to the earth, your mother. Take another deep breath and gently open your eyes.[1]

Why Energy Medicine Today?

Today there is a surge in curiosity about energy-based medicine, which I believe is primarily due to society's needs going largely unmet by our medical system. Many people will agree that the present health-care system is in many respects broken. Did you know, for example, that *hospitalization* is a leading cause of death in the U.S. and other countries? What was meant to heal is actually causing harm in staggering numbers. Less publicized is that cancer is not only *not* being eradicated, but it is actually increasing exponentially, everywhere.

Our modern medical system also doesn't address the whole person, which leaves us dissatisfied, even if unconsciously. It doesn't concentrate on the underlying causes of disease, and therefore it doesn't treat them. This is one of the reasons why energy medicine is so valuable: it goes beyond just the body, including the psychological and spiritual dimensions as well.

Energy Medicine at Work

Let me give you an example to illustrate energy medicine at work. A woman named Carol joined me at the front of the room in one of my energy healing workshops and told me she was dealing with breast cancer. She'd already had a lumpectomy and radiation and was still undergoing chemotherapy. She'd come to the event

---

[1]*Ancient Shamanic Meditation Through the Chakras,* a guided meditation CD by Deborah King, takes you on a magical journey through the hidden realms of your energy field and beyond, promoting inner peace, otherworldly wisdom, and spiritual advancement. Please visit **www.deborahkingcenter.com/ChakraMeditationCD** or call 800-790-5785 for more information.

to find out what else she could do to recover. First, I sensed into Carol's body and energy field, where I discerned a great deal of anger, guilt, and remorse—a potent stew of emotions that would make anyone sick. I asked her if someone close to her had recently died. She answered that, yes, her mother, with whom she'd had a difficult relationship, had passed a few years before.

Initially, I perceived that the combination of surgery, radiation, and chemo had caused Carol's first chakra to stop spinning. A first chakra that is shut down means that the individual won't be able to connect to Mother Earth, the very source of physical healing. This is a pretty common response to such aggressive and invasive, though often lifesaving, treatments. Fortunately, energy medicine can help ameliorate unwanted side effects of traditional therapies such as these, while still preserving their beneficial effects.

Finally, I observed in Carol's energy field that her third chakra was circling the wrong way. It was in a state of inward collapse and looked like a truck had run over it—her mother's controlling and overpowering personality had left her with a "flattened" sense of self. Additionally, Carol's fourth chakra, the energy center of the heart, was completely shut down in an effort to avoid feeling her mother's constant rejection. Carol also had a daughter from whom she was estranged—a mirror of what she had experienced with her own mother—and this was one more reason to close her heart to all feeling.

As you have just learned, problems show up first in our energy field and only later manifest in the body. Unless Carol worked to release her pain and the guilt she felt about not being a good enough daughter and mother—even if she had a remission—she might very well find herself dealing with a recurrence of the cancer within a few short years.

I began Carol's healing by balancing and charging her energy field and chakras and connecting her base chakra directly to the earth. Then, joining deeply with the universal energy field, I attracted its power and transmitted it to Carol, conducting it through my own field and body first. This universal energy is of a higher vibration, and its laserlike intensity jump-started Carol's healing by eliminating the stored emotions that had caused the cancer in the first place. I also cleared out the anesthetics and chemo I found in her body and energy field. Last, I disconnected Carol from the negative energy drain of her mother (still in place after death, as death does not separate us energetically) so that her sense of self-esteem could be rebuilt.

Following the healing work, I recommended that Carol take up the practice of journaling to get more in touch with her emotions and provide a safe place to release her guilt and remorse, as well as the fear and other feelings that came up during surgery and chemo. In order to heal and open up to the possibility of happiness, she would have to stop blaming herself.

I heard from Carol some months later. She reported that she felt a lot less fearful immediately after our session and had started sleeping more and berating herself less. She said that her oncologist was very pleased with her progress and had cancelled a possible second round of chemo. In response to a suggestion I had made for her to get a pet, she had adopted a new puppy and was delighting in his company. Pets, with their tremendous ability for unconditional love, help us reopen our heart chakras.

By zeroing in on the root cause of a disease, blasting away the emotions that created it in the first place, and offering continued support in the form of tools for self-healing, energy medicine paves the way for the body to heal itself. Its ability to do so is a basic tenet of this practice, with practitioners to facilitate the process.

All Hands on Deck, with You at the Helm

Because energy medicine can address root causes, it can help you clear toxic emotions you may not even realize you have. Often, these feelings stem from childhood experiences that are, thank goodness, repressed. It's important to know that it isn't essential to recall anything that was repressed. Indeed, it's not *safe* to try to remember. All that's necessary to heal from something that happened to you, no matter how long ago it was, is to deal with what you're feeling today. If you're currently struggling with health issues, energy healing helps you focus on those underlying emotions and clear them.

Energy medicine balances your energy and removes blockages, which then allows standard medical practices, like chemotherapy, to work more efficiently; and conversely, as we saw in the example of Carol, it can also remove these chemicals from the body after they have done their work, thus reducing the body's toxic load. I have seen many people sail through chemo with no side effects because they received energy-medicine treatments at the same time.

Advocates on either side of the dispute between traditional and alternative medicine often wholly discount each other's value. It has been my experience that by the time a problem has festered to the point that a disease is diagnosed, an aggressive and collaborative effort is needed to ensure healing. "All hands on deck" may be required to remove the illness: a surgeon and oncologist, if necessary; a medical specialist to offer treatment options; an acupuncturist to help maintain balance; a nutritionist to build strength and decrease toxins; and a practitioner of energy medicine to address the core issues so that the disease is cured at the root and won't return.

When working to heal serious illnesses, it is imperative to treat the cause of the problem, not merely the symptoms. Any work that is directed toward healing our wounded minds and spirits allows our bodies to open up and receive the benefits of conventional medicine. With energy medicine, we create a clearer energy flow, which strengthens the body. With a stronger body, we achieve an even greater energy flow, and thus a more balanced spirit and mind. It becomes a positive cycle of healing.

Here's the bottom line: If you're ill, leave no stone unturned—get everyone on your team. But remember that you are the director of that team, in charge of what happens to you. While conventional allopathic medicine focuses on the physical treatment of disease, complementary and alternative modalities offer other benefits.

I encourage you to listen closely to the diagnosis (but not necessarily the prognosis!) of conventional medicine. I also urge you to learn to use your intuition about the best course of treatment *for you,* and that's really what this book is all about—developing your abilities and intuition. Your opinion should carry the most significant weight in the decision-making process. So many people feel disempowered by the medical establishment and its "authorities" and "experts." I want to put the patient back in the driver's seat.

If you have a problem, whether it's spiritual, emotional, or physical, you are the ultimate arbiter of the solution. If you've been given a diagnosis of cancer, for instance, you may very well want to include any number of different avenues in your approach to wellness, from surgery and/or chemo combined with nutrition and counseling, to energy work to eradicate the original cause, ameliorate the effects of the chemo, and boost your immune system. These are all completely valid approaches. Someone else might just want whatever the doctor recommends plus an occasional massage. That's okay, too. Every person is different.

Your solution could also be the exact opposite of the medical recommendations. The important thing is that you take back your power and not bow down in acquiescence to the first words out of a physician's mouth. You have the right to be a vocal part of the process and be aware of all the tools available to help you lead a happy, healthy, and successful life. You, in the deepest part of your heart, know what's right for you.

As a healer, you give people a valuable gift when you help them get past their fear and assist them in making the right decision for their own care. I often counsel people to have the surgery that they're fearing, or I simply attempt to help clear their confusion that stems from getting two or three separate, and possibly conflicting, opinions.

Fear really does hold us back. So often it's this emotion, or people feeling that they don't have the right to make decisions on their own, that holds them back from getting the care they need. One gentleman I worked with, a charming man of about

75, had a life-threatening hernia. Hernias can get extremely serious if you ignore them, and he was at that point. He was against the proposed surgery because of a fear of anesthesia, but it was clear to me as I listened to him—at the level below his personality where all of the fear was rooted—that his higher self thought that it was the right option. I helped him clear this negative emotion and encouraged him to make the decision to go through with the surgery. In the end, he was very appreciative. The procedure was a success, and the anesthesia was not a problem.

As a beginner in this wonderful field of energy medicine, you are your very own first client. You will use the principles offered here to optimize your body's natural healing abilities. It won't be long before you notice that nagging problems, such as insomnia or anxiety or poor digestion or a little depression, begin to disappear as you naturally move into a state of self-healing. And should you begin to practice your skills on others, that same self-healing mechanism will continue to operate.

Before you can heal anyone though, you'll need some information that has to come from a very trustworthy source. The next chapter will guide you in expanding your consciousness so that you can access the greatest possible source of knowledge about healing: *the unified field.*

chapter two

EXPANDING YOUR CONSCIOUSNESS

To heal ourselves and others, we need information. We need to get to the bottom—to the root cause—of our illnesses and pain, whether it's physical, emotional, or spiritual. And we need to find out what the most efficient and effective means of healing will be for each of us individually.

We get information about ourselves and our environment in two very different ways: One is through our normal five senses— sight, sound, touch, taste, and smell. The other is through an expanded state of awareness, where we perceive beyond the limitations of our body and mind and feel that we are part of the vast universe around us, connected to All That Is. In this state, we have access to unlimited information.

Perhaps you have had such an experience while hiking in the mountains or watching the waves roll in at the beach—nature can certainly ease you into an expanded state of awareness. Or maybe you've reached it through exercise or prayer or music, or through making love or being present at the birth or death of a loved one— events where you felt deeply connected to another person. Please keep in mind that I'm referring to *naturally* expanded states, not ones of artificial expansion from drugs, which can damage the human energy field, sometimes permanently.

Oftentimes, an expanded state has come upon me while mountain climbing or cross-country skiing in the wilderness. But the surest route to heightened consciousness is meditation.

I was once on a yearlong meditation retreat with a spiritual teacher, receiving instruction in ancient Hindu *sutras,* which are highly condensed texts (usually short phrases or even single words) that are memorized in order to produce specific effects. Students are instructed to focus on these sutras while meditating. Having been admitted to the program at the 11th hour, I'd had no opportunity to read books or quiz friends as to what I could expect. And since the 200 students were instructed not to discuss the sutras among themselves, I simply showed up each day ready to sit silently and await instruction.

Once the last sutra had been whispered to me, I began quietly repeating it in my mind. Suddenly, I noticed my whole body become very hot, as if it were on fire. The heat became more and more intense, and I began to vibrate—just a little at first, and then a great deal. I felt my body expand . . . and expand . . . and expand . . . until it seemed that there were no longer 200 separate people sitting on the floor, but one vast body. It was as if we were so linked that we were all one, beating with one heart. Although I didn't know it at the time, I had, for a brief moment, experienced the unified field, where we are all intimately connected.

Once you have experienced a direct connection to this energy, you will not want to live without it. It truly feels like home.

The Source of All Information

Why would you want to cultivate expanded consciousness? Besides the fact that it feels really good, it's also the best state from which to get guidance and direction for your life, to have your energy field recharged (resulting in better health), and to get the information and instructions you need for healing. All of the concerns that your "small self" doesn't know how to address, as well as all of your bigger life questions, can be answered by tapping into this unlimited field. Being in an expanded state allows you to connect to your own highest qualities and the field of all possibilities. If you stay only in your little mind all of the time, separated from this source, you're not allowing yourself to connect to the vastness of information that lies just beyond it.

Many of the most brilliant thinkers in human history have reported that they received their biggest insights after meditating, napping, or being in a state of reverie. Among them was Newton's crucial discovery of the principle of gravity. He was reportedly meandering through a garden in a contemplative state when he saw an apple fall from a tree and the notion of gravity came into his mind. Evidently, he had tapped into the unified field.

In energy medicine, it's vital that you're able to go into an expanded state of consciousness easily and at will. All of the knowledge and power you need to effect change in yourself and others is out there, right beyond your everyday senses. When you are able to access the unified field intentionally, you have the ability to discover anything in the universe—past, present, or future. And this information can be the basis of your helping others achieve transformation in their lives, which is the very foundation of energy medicine.

The more expanded your consciousness, the more your extrasensory perceptions will increase, the more you will be able to access and see beyond this plane, and the more valid the information you receive will be. Ultimately, with training, you'll be able to attract the power of that infinite field of energy for yourself, and even conduct and transmit it to others.

As I've described, I mastered going into an expanded state in my childhood quite inadvertently, as I spent time there every day in prayer, communing with nature, and keeping all of my senses attuned to the possibility of parental abuse. Later, as a young adult, I learned how to connect intentionally to that same state with meditation, prayer, and working on healing both myself and others. I'm always amazed by how easily information comes from the unified field. That is, it comes easily if you don't *try* to get it; if you make too much of an effort, you'll get nothing, or nothing real. Instead, simply be open and receptive, and what you need will come to you.

What happens when you meditate correctly and regularly for some time is that eventually your brain begins to function in a much more coherent way, which allows you to access intelligence that is beyond regular waking consciousness. The more you meditate, the more information will come to you, and you can really rely on its accuracy. (We'll be delving into meditation in greater depth later in this book.)

For many years I would enter an expanded state every time I meditated, prayed, or worked in a healing environment; and then for the rest of the day I'd go back to everyday consciousness. I found it too exhausting to stay "wide open" during my regular business day—there's just so much information that comes in when you're in that state! But when I left the corporate world, I quit the back-and-forth and simply remained expanded. Now *that* feels normal to me, and each day I work to expand further. Remember, the unified field is limitless, which means that there is no end to how expanded any of us can be.

And I haven't even mentioned all of the other benefits that come from an expanded state of consciousness, such as peace, joy, deep rest, and better health!

EXERCISE: Your Consciousness as a Computer

Imagine for a moment that your consciousness is a computer, similar to the one on your desk. Day to day, this machine performs millions of tasks per second, just as your brain does. Now consider that, out there in the great unified field of all knowledge—which, for this metaphor, I'll call the World Wide Web—are all of the bits and bytes of information you could ever need or want to gather. This means anything and everything, from whether that guy or gal is the right one for you, to the highest wisdom of the saints and sages. And it all exists in complete accuracy on this infinite World Wide Web.

How does your computer access the Web? Well, first it must connect, either through an Ethernet or wirelessly; and then it must expand its reach, which it does through a search engine. Meditation would be your device for these tasks. Practices such as meditation and prayer take you beyond the database of your ordinary senses and memory so you can "search" for the advanced knowledge and guidance you seek. Your expanded consciousness gives you the ability to connect and search beyond the rational workings of your hard-drive mind. When you access this vast scope of "cyberspace," you receive messages from the universe that you need to hear for your continued growth and evolution.

The more expanded your consciousness, the greater your ability to access and see beyond this physical plane—beyond the ordinary nuts and bolts of life—and the more valid the information will be that you'll get for yourself and, ultimately, for others.

To begin tapping into the unified field and obtaining answers to your questions, try utilizing the following process:

1. Take a moment now to begin thinking about a few of the questions you have for the unified field.

2. Write down these questions and state your intent to receive the answers.

3. As you continue reading through this book, exploring the various pathways and clues it offers, make notes of any relevant insights you receive that begin to answer your questions.

Change Your Dreams to Change Your Life

There are four major states of consciousness: *waking, sleeping, dreaming,* and *meditative* (called *contemplative* in the West). If you meditate every day, correctly and consistently, you will soon find that it affects the other states. For example, after I had been meditating for a few years, I noticed that I needed less sleep. After a few more years, I realized that I had begun dreaming in a much more directed way. As more time went by, I felt as if I were in a state of meditation all the time, floating between states of consciousness, often above my body.

Waking consciousness is our day-to-day awareness. It is how we function in the world and where we live most of the time when we're not asleep. Dreaming gives us access to subconscious thoughts and feelings. Keeping a dream journal is a good way to see what our unconscious considers important, and it can be a valuable source of information to help in the healing process.

The dream state can also open a window into a more expanded consciousness through the process of *lucid dreaming*, in which one can actually change the outcomes of one's dreams. This means that the sleeper is aware that he or she is dreaming and can actively participate in and manipulate what is experienced in the dream.

In one of my own lucid dreams, my entire family, including my mother, was standing in front of a giant display of my last book, *Truth Heals*, looking quite unhappy. If you've read it, you know that I basically aired my family's dirty laundry. Because I wanted them to be comfortable with the publication of the material, I used my lucid dream to change their reaction to it. While in this state, I simply formed the conscious intent—the thought about what I desired—to have them feel positive about the book. The next thing I knew, my family started to smile and congratulate me on its success. Although the dream started one way, I was able to change the outcome to one that I desired. Then, sure enough, after that dream, I noticed that my family members seemed much more at peace with the book being published.

All of the ancients knew that the dream of life and our nightly dreams are very much alike, although we are more attached to the seemingly "real" forms of waking life. With lucid dreaming, living may seem more like a dream, while the dream may feel far more alive.

The primary aim of this practice is to realize that you're dreaming while still in the dream. Then you can do all sorts of beneficial things, such as receive initiations and special powers, which are exciting spiritual "steps up" that we will be discussing later in this book. For example, in one lucid dream that came to me following an especially deep meditation, I received the power to energetically raise entire groups of people to a higher plane, where each individual feels an expansion in his or her consciousness.

In a lucid dream, you can also go to different places, even different planes; you can communicate with the dead and with spirits; you can even fly and shape-shift, changing your own form as needed for a particular realm. I have the firm intention to learn through lucid dreaming how to bilocate in this lifetime—imagine how convenient it would be for me to speak in Los Angeles and Munich on the same day!

Past Lives

Each of us can access information by going into an expanded state of consciousness through many different pathways. Another source of information that is occasionally helpful in solving the mystery of where certain pain, disease, or other dysfunction stem from involves exploration of our past lives.

Past lives refer to *reincarnation,* which means "to be made flesh again" or "transmigration of the soul." It describes how, after the body dies, the soul or spirit of a person survives and comes back to Earth in the body of a newborn to live anew. It's only here in the West that reincarnation is not a commonly shared belief, as it is in the remaining two-thirds of the world. If you want to study the scientific basis of reincarnation, you can find it best described in ancient Hindu texts.

I've done healings for thousands of people, and sometimes information from past lives will surface. There are certain levels of the human energy field that allow us easier access to a person's past lives. I will put myself on one of those levels whenever I can't find the source for someone's problems in *this* life. I was working with a 50-year-old man named Larry, for instance, who complained of a terrible pain in his upper back that had plagued him since he was a teenager. Nothing helped—not massage, not manual osteopathy, not acupuncture, not even pain pills. I went to the fifth level of his human energy field and found a knife stuck in his back that had been the cause of his death in a former lifetime. Once I energetically removed the weapon, Larry's suffering went away.

My own past-life memories are quite vivid. At one point in my spiritual practice, I had extended my meditation time to four hours a day, as I was trying to master the lost art of instantaneous healing and had a hunch that this would give me a portal into that arena. What I didn't count on was that it would also open a door into my past lives. I would be floating along in, say, the third hour of meditation, when all of a sudden I'd be transported to a completely different era. I had many meditations where I found myself working in what felt like an underground temple in ancient Egypt. I, along with the other spiritual adepts, would be wearing what looked like a uniform. We all seemed quite young, perhaps around 15 years old. I remember learning how to levitate there—a paranormal skill I'm still working on in this lifetime!

In a much more unpleasant experience, I remembered being burned at the stake. Perhaps that's why I feel so strongly about helping women (and men) who have been unjustly treated in some way. Later, I had meditations where I was the abbess at a convent in charge of the other nuns. To this day, anytime I go into a chapel or convent, I feel right at home.

I have one important note of caution about delving into your past lives: the only way you can change your karma is to change yourself in *this* lifetime. People get too hung up on what may or may not have transpired in a past life. It is certainly fun and entertaining, but never forget that the only life you have is the one you are experiencing today, and it's in this one that you want to effect change. You do so by clearing past traumas and releasing blocked energy. And reading this book has already put you on that path.

Dowsing with a Pendulum

Another great tool for receiving information that isn't available through the normal five senses is dowsing with a pendulum. A pendulum is a simple object that's suspended by a cord, and it increases your sensitivity to energy flow by acting as an amplifier. It helps you access the unified field, as well as your higher self—the part of you that extends beyond your first seven chakras and houses your highest attributes, such as vision, courage, integrity, and steadfastness.

Pendulums have been employed for divination for thousands of years. Among their well-known users were the ancient Romans and the famous French seer Nostradamus. These folks would hold the pendulum over a basin that had the characters of the Greek alphabet inscribed on it and allow its movement to spell out answers to their questions. In addition to getting information from your unconscious, this tool will help you ascertain the location and activity of a chakra. You can then use the feedback to confirm the information you get in sensing chakras with your hands, body, or energy field.

I counsel against the use of metal or crystal pendulums when you're just starting out, since they take quite of bit of training to use properly, and require a higher level of consciousness from the operator. A crystal also has a strong field of its own that can distort the fields around it. When you're learning, you'll want to use a wood pendulum (preferably beech) with a conical shape, which is best for giving you the information you're looking for without interference from other energy fields. You'll find a website in the Appendix where you can get information about some pendulums made of beech that are just right for this purpose. When you first get your pendulum, carry it around with you for a few days in a little pouch or your pocket so it begins to resonate with your energy.

Everyone is capable of working with a pendulum, but it does require practice—much like learning to play a musical instrument.

EXERCISE: Using a Pendulum to
Get Information from Your Unconscious

The first step in using your pendulum is to bless it. You'll want to do this before each and every use. I might affirm, for example, that I want my higher self and the higher beings that are prepared to assist me (you'll learn about these in a moment) to influence the movement of the pendulum.

Then, hold the cord between the thumb and forefinger of your dominant hand (that is, if you're right-handed, use your right hand), with your elbow resting on a table, the arm of a chair, or your knee so it can dangle freely. Keep your hand and arm completely still. When the pendulum stops moving, you're ready to ask a question. Note that working with a pendulum requires you to ask questions where the answer can only be "Yes" or "No."

To get started, ask a question to which you know the answer is "Yes." For example, I would ask, "Is my name Deborah?" Pay attention to which way the pendulum begins to move—side to side, clockwise, or counterclockwise. This direction of movement will always signify "Yes" to you. Test several questions where you know for sure that they have "Yes" answers and verify that the movement remains the same. Do the same thing with some inquiries where you know that the answer is "No." Looking for a "No" answer, I might ask, "Is my name Doug?" and then record the direction of that movement. Perform this test as much as you need to until a clear pattern emerges.

Now you're ready to start asking questions that your personality and conscious mind don't know the answers to, but your unconscious and higher self do. This isn't magic, although it may seem like it; rather, it's a way of accessing the part of you that is connected to the unified field and, therefore, wiser and more knowledgeable than your everyday consciousness. Be sure to phrase your questions very clearly and with specificity. "Am I going to have a relationship?" is too vague. Instead, you'll want to ask, "Am I going to have a relationship with Zachary, the man I met in line at Starbucks an hour ago?" Notice how I narrowed down the scope of the question.

When using a pendulum, you'll want to center yourself and relax. Focus only on the question you're asking so that you don't accidentally influence your results with an answer you want. That is, clear your mind of any expectations. Doing this is the hardest part of the whole process; you need to relax and become quiet inside.

Once you've become comfortable with the pendulum, you can use it to check someone else's chakras or energy centers. Here's a quick reminder of where the chakras are located:

- *First Chakra:* behind the genitals
- *Second Chakra:* halfway between the first chakra and the waist
- *Third Chakra:* halfway between the navel and the breastbone
- *Fourth Chakra:* in the center of the chest
- *Fifth Chakra:* in the center of the throat
- *Sixth Chakra:* between the eyebrows
- *Seventh Chakra:* at the top of the head

EXERCISE: Testing Chakras With a Pendulum

Begin by having your subject lie down on her back, preferably on a surface that is at a height where you can maintain a straight and comfortable posture. You don't want to be leaning into the person, which is referred to as being *on push,* where your own energy is being pushed into hers.

With your posture straight and your arm extended forward from your body, suspend the pendulum over each energy center, about four to six inches above the chakras. As the pendulum starts to move, note the direction of its movement. Is it clockwise, counterclockwise, elliptical, or not moving at all? Write this down, and then move up to the next chakra.

Note the following:

- *Clockwise* movement indicates that the chakra is open and the feelings governed by it are well balanced and full.

- *Counterclockwise* movement indicates possible blocked energy or negative experiences with the feelings related to that chakra. Whether the circle is larger or smaller also tells us, respectively, whether the energy is flowing nicely or restricted.

- An *elliptical* swing indicates a right- or left-side imbalance of energy flow in the body, perhaps due to overusing either the right masculine side or the left nurturing side.

- *No movement at all* can indicate that you're holding the pendulum above the wrong place on the body or, if you are in the correct location, blockage.

Here's a key point to remember: the size of the chakra is not the size of the circle that the pendulum makes; rather, the size of the pendulum's circle is a function of your energy field combined with both that of the pendulum and the subject. So the health of your own field has a direct impact on your effectiveness in reading the other person's energy centers. With practice, you'll be able to pick up qualities of each chakra, such as joy, peace, or clarity; or heaviness, darkness, or grief.

Don't be discouraged if, when you first begin, you find that you can't even figure out where the chakras are. Practice, practice, practice. It won't be long before you'll start to see results.

For the maintenance of your pendulum, every full moon (without heavy moisture) place it outside in the moonlight in order for it to clear and recharge. Also, it's best not to loan your pendulum to others unless it's for the purpose of testing your own chakras.

Locating Your Spirit Guides

A wonderful source of information from the unified field is spirit guides. All of us have beings on the inner planes who are waiting to help us obtain the answers we want or need. The guides and mentors in the invisible realms are specific to each individual's personal beliefs and spiritual lineage. For some, a revered ancestor or power animal, such as an eagle or bear, may have the most significance. Others may orient to an enlightened person, living or deceased: one or more of the pantheon of Hindu or Tibetan deities; Buddha; or the energy of Jesus, referred to as the *Christ light.*

Connecting to your various guides will provide you with a great way to expand your power and access to information.

EXERCISE: Connecting to Your Ancestral Guides

When we're not aware of our guides, it doesn't mean that they don't exist or have deserted us; we simply fail to recognize their presence. We all have relatives, some recent and some way back in our family tree, who are ready, willing, and able to give us help—all we have to do is ask them. There's absolutely no reason to go it alone.

The following steps will help you connect to an ancestral guide who is there for you. Among the most common of these guides are deceased grandparents, but use your intuition in choosing your ancestor—it could be anyone in your family tree.

1. When you go to bed at night, after you turn out the light and before you fall asleep, state (out loud or silently) your intention to connect to whatever ancestor is most available to you.

2. Choose the person, whether or not you knew him or her personally, who resonates with you the most. Chances are, whoever first comes to your mind is the right one.

3. Picture your ancestor in whatever form most appeals to you.

4. Tell this individual that you want him or her to be there for you. Ask this spirit a specific question or for help with a particular problem. You may very well see this guide later in your dreams.

Don't discount what your dead relatives can do for you from the Other Side simply because they had an imperfect life. Who didn't?! One of my guides is my grandfather, whom I was close to as a child, and he had all sorts of personal problems. He was a binge drinker and kept losing his job as a fireman, but somewhere along the way he must have cleaned up his act, perhaps during his last very painful and frightening illness. All I know is that when he comes through to me now, he feels very . . . not "high up there," but not in the darkness either. My grandfather seems interested in my welfare, ready and able to help. Somehow he straightened out his karma, and he is quite a strong guide for me in certain areas of my life. I call upon him when I'm lost, whether in the mountains hiking or on a freeway where I can't find the correct exit. He was evidently really good with maps and compasses, because whenever I ask him for assistance, he points me in the right direction.

The information you'll get from your guides is only as good as their connection to Source. For example, I'd ask my grandfather for help with a practical problem or a family issue, but I wouldn't request his help to effect healing in others. That might very well be beyond his current level of consciousness. So chances are you will be using your deceased relatives and the people in your family lineage as guides for the practical things in your life.

In addition to ancestors, you can also access experts who have passed on. From South American shamans, I learned how to connect with deceased physicians, to do etheric template surgery (which is discussed later in Chapter 8). If you're taking an exam or doing a project in a specific field of study, you can access the energy of a noted scholar who was prominent in that subject and ask for assistance.

These opportunities are always available to us. As we've learned, we are all connected at the level of the unified field. We in the West are probably the only culture in history that doesn't know how to utilize the talents and willing assistance of those who have come before us.

Here is the main rule to remember with guides: they want to help, but they won't *unless they are specifically asked.*

When I work with volunteers from the audience at workshops or other events, I can invariably sense that their guides are standing nearby. I'll inquire, "Are you connected to your guides?"

"What guides?" they'll often ask.

"Well, you've got all of these people around you; there's actually one just off your left shoulder who's dying to help. It feels like your uncle [or grandmother, or someone in his or her lineage]."

Or I'll say, "Archangel Michael is big in your energy field. Did you know that?"

A typical response is, "Not really, but I always hoped I was connected to him."

If you just take a few moments every day, in the morning and at night, to tune in to your guides, you can ask them exactly what you want assistance with, and they will be more than happy to comply.

You may also be able to step up another level energetically by working with a being on the Other Side who was incredibly advanced spiritually and had a matching energy field while here on Earth—someone like Jesus, Buddha, or one of the great Tibetan or Indian masters.

Still another level of guidance comes to us from the angelic realm. Angels are advanced energy forms that we anthropomorphize (give human qualities to), but they have never lived as a human on Earth. For example, Archangel Michael isn't really a person—he never actually lived—but he's an energy that many of us can sense and have given a name; and artists have given us images of him as a male being with enormous wings.

What's interesting about working with guides is that when you become more attuned and have developed your extrasensory abilities enough, you can really tell the difference between them. The distinction is palpable and very real. You can learn to discern between the energy of a deceased physician and, say, that of the Madonna, the energy that was incarnated as Jesus's mother, Mary. It's like comparing your desktop computer to the giant network of computers of an international company. The energy fields feel dramatically unlike each other.

A large energy field, by the way, can knock you right off your feet. The time I was present for an apparition of the Madonna (more about that amazing experience later), I was literally thrown to my knees. Now, 15 years later, I'm able to connect to her energy as well as attract, conduct, and transmit it through my body to others for healing. Over the years and because of all the work I've done, my field has been recalibrated to withstand her energy. Yours can be, too!

An important side note I'd like to bring up here is that when I talk about the Madonna, I'm referring to the archetype of the Divine Feminine that has surfaced in many living individuals throughout the ages. One of her earliest appearances was as Isis, the Egyptian goddess. The most recent manifestations have been as the Virgin Mary, both in her actual lifetime and her many subsequent visitations as Our Lady of Lourdes, Our Lady at Fátima,

Our Lady of Guadalupe, and the Black Madonna (as statues or paintings of Mary with European features and dark skin found all over the world that have been associated with more than a few miracles).

And just as the Madonna is much more than a figure in the story of one particular religion, Jesus is not only the basis for the Christian religion, but also a spirit guide and a manifestation of the archetype known as the Christ light.

Meditation, dreams, past lives, pendulums, and spirit guides—as we've seen, there is a wide variety of ways to access the information held in the unified and human energy fields. This chapter illustrates only a few. When we are able to connect to these forces, we can receive the information we need to heal ourselves and the clues necessary to help others. We have the ability to get the answers to questions that baffle us, and solutions to our problems. We can hear the whispers of our higher self and our guides, and learn to trust in the wisdom of the universe as well as that which lies within ourselves.

To further develop confidence in our place in the lineage of great healers, we'll explore a bit of the history of healing in the next chapter.

chapter three

HEALING THROUGHOUT THE AGES

Long ago in human history, when science and religion were one and a shaman led our little band (and that shaman was often a woman), we could see others' energy fields as well as the energy fields of the plants and animals that shared our world. We had the ability, as I've mentioned, to communicate telepathically with other humans, other living things on the planet, and our ancestors; and we were very connected to spirit, our Source. All of us had at least some familiarity with the basic concepts of energy medicine—that our energy fields are healing instruments—and some of us became quite adept at healing.

In most societies that flourished before the written word, the gods were female. Amazed by women's ability to give birth, our ancestors projected godlike powers onto them. Healing was their natural domain; they were the midwives and the first caregivers. And that caregiver-patient relationship likely continued after the birth of a baby, since the bond between midwife, mother, and child ensured survival of the species. This laid the foundation for healing and medicine.

James Cameron, the writer, director, and producer of the amazing film *Avatar,* obviously plugged into the unified field of consciousness to create the mystical land of Pandora and the Na'vi tribe when he made this film. It's the closest depiction I can imagine to the world I see and the way I feel when I am actively engaged in healing work.

We all share the ancient, innate capacities of the Na'vi. We crave their reality, just like we crave the sea, because it's where we once came from. Everyone in the Na'vi clan is connected energetically, and they manifest healing power through their rituals. It's no accident that the most powerful person in their world is a female shaman, a representation of the Divine Feminine. Today, as women return to the forefront of shamanism, they are making that fictional depiction a reality.

The Ancients

Every ancient culture on Earth, from the Mayan and the Aztec to the East Indian and Chinese, had healing systems that worked with the human energy field. In these societies, the role of priest and healer was unified under the term *shaman.* Medicinal plants and prayer were important in treatment, and Divine intervention was considered essential. Europeans of the same time period, however, had a much more primitive understanding of these practices.

About 6,000 years ago in Mesopotamia—the area of present-day Iraq—the Sumerians laid the foundation for what we experience today in the West as modern healing. This civilization was very advanced in math, writing, architecture, astronomy, and medicine.

With the advent of the alphabet in Egyptian society (about 2,000 B.C.), men eventually replaced women as the chief healers. It's likely that the development of the written word led us away from being balanced between our masculine left brain and feminine right brain to the point where we are today: a society of warmongering, left-brained people. Please don't get me wrong—I'm

36

not knocking men. Rather, it's the masculine side we all have, women as well as men, that has become too dominant.

It was the Greeks who were said to have begun the formal study of medicine, distinct from religion, with the Hippocratic school of thought. Both the Greeks and the Jews believed in a split between the mind and the body, and saw the body as evil. For the Greeks, sickness indicated disfavor from the gods and was seen as a matter of luck or fate. The Judaic view, on the other hand, regarded sickness as a punishment for sin, which became a pervasive theme in Judaic teachings in the form of plagues, fevers, madness, leprosy, and so on. In both cultures, only the Greek gods or Yahweh could intervene and bring about healing. Although doctors were sought out to mitigate illness, the art they practiced was considered magic and, therefore, suspect.

This low regard for the body led to a lack of appreciation for healing, and even for practices that would lead to better health. There is still much of this mind-set running through today's collective unconscious. Check into your own thoughts the next time you're sick; you may very well hear that you're ill because you've somehow been bad. This unconscious belief, incidentally, could be an important reason why some people don't heal.

Jesus, the Master Healer

At about the same time that the belief that disease was caused by sin was in vogue, Jesus Christ, the man, entered the world stage. He exploded onto the healing scene, setting the bar so high that no one has matched it since. After all, he was way ahead of his time . . . around 2,000 years! Somehow, he jumped from the reality of his era—a first-chakra era of physical power and kill or be killed—to the age we're just stepping into. In the Aquarian Age, we'll be centered in a fourth-chakra, or heart-centered, reality.

Jesus's healing ministry represented a radical departure from the prevailing ideology of his time. His critical point of difference from the Greek and Hebrew worldviews to which he was born was his belief that sickness was not punishment for sins and did not indicate disfavor from God. In the Jewish belief system, very occasionally God was said to intervene and cause a healing. With Jesus, this concept was turned upside down: his miraculous healings were revolutionary because he was a man, not a god. So vast a departure was he from what was understood at the time that he was accused of doing the work of the devil. However, his detractors never denied that he did, in fact, effect profound healings.

Although Jesus was also well known for his preaching and teaching, his healing demonstrations received the most attention by far. To that end, about a fifth of the New Testament is devoted to recording these events. More than 40 distinct instances were recorded, many of which involved healing large crowds of people (a much more difficult achievement, by the way, than walking on water, which only involves one's own energy field as opposed to those of a crowd of people). Everywhere he went, groups gathered in the hopes of being healed. In fact, the principal reason for the spread of Christ's name was this healing work.

During his brief time on Earth, Jesus consistently emphasized compassion and care. The cornerstone of his message was the power of love. Somehow, he had managed to open his chakras a full 360 degrees. If we could open our chakras that completely, we, too, would be able to do things like change water into wine, heal the multitudes, and physically ascend from this plane to the next.

The Christ energy, or Christ light, evolved from Jesus's fully opened chakras and what psychologist Abraham Maslow would call his fully self-actualized personality. That's the energy that those of us who want to heal others strive to merge with so closely that we won't be able to distinguish where our fields end and his begins. Think of that light as the ancestral Source that we are connecting to—a white light that illuminates us, heals all, and holds the secret to instantaneous transformations.

In his sophisticated comprehension of psychology, Jesus understood the power of evil and knew that the human personality was susceptible to its influence. He realized that these dark forces could manipulate our behavior—a view that didn't become widely accepted in the West until the early 1900s during the time of Carl Jung. Jesus never passed judgment or talked about sin. He simply treated everyone with love, which was a remarkable act at a time when very little was known about the mechanics of healing and disease.

He told his followers to do exactly as he had done: go out and heal. And they did. In those early days, Christ's followers lived in an environment where daily healings were expected. For some 300 years after his death, they performed what were called "signs and wonders" in his name. They emulated Jesus, moving from an aware and open heart as he had, to do all they could to relieve suffering. When you heal from an open heart, it works.

So where did Jesus learn his skills? Ancient cultures before his time understood that it was possible for one individual to mediate with the unseen world on behalf of others. In other words, thousands of years before the birth of Christ, shamans acted as instruments of grace.

Some of the masters I've studied with believe that Jesus spent time with the Essenes, an esoteric group of spiritual adepts who likely had a secret society and carried with them the knowledge of healing that was forbidden by the authorities. It's very possible that Jesus was a member of this brotherhood and received early training from them. The more you study the history of healing, the more likely it will seem that he was exposed to these teachings. (There are many stories in India of his having spent time there with great masters, too.)

Another possibility is that Jesus was simply able to access the information he needed to effect instantaneous healings by expanding his awareness and retrieving it from the unified field. I am convinced that we will be able to duplicate this master healer's work in our times. I believe that the current level of consciousness —which you are raising just by reading this book—combined with our level of world crisis, offers the perfect set of circumstances to reproduce his achievements.

After Jesus

In the early Christian church, special healing skills and rituals were initially the province of women. As you can imagine, that was a very brief period. It's likely that by about a century after Jesus's death, women had been completely pushed into the background. From that point on, only the Pope and his bishops were allowed to harness these powers, and priests were selected for advancement on the basis of their spiritual aptitude and self-mastery.

If we look at the original meaning and intent of the sacraments, each can clearly be viewed as an initiatory rite that was specifically designed to mark a passage into a new state of consciousness and open the aspirant to the next level of development. When a child is baptized, he becomes a watermarked member of the tribe. At First Communion, he becomes energetically connected with the founder of the group, Jesus Christ. Confirmation is another ritual where the bishop, with the power to bring down the Holy Spirit, anoints him with holy oil. Then, if he chooses to become ordained as a priest, he steps up to the plate to become a healer, just like the man he follows. So far, so good.

Unfortunately, perhaps 300 years after the death of Jesus, the clergy lost its way, its members overcome by their own egos. *Remember, pride is the nemesis of every healer.* The church leaders lost the ability to transmit the "gifts of the spirit" and heal, and their ceremonies became nothing but hollow ritual. What are these "gifts" that were commemorated in the sacraments? They are the very same abilities and skills I teach and devote a chapter to later in this book.

Within 400 or 500 years after Jesus's death, the Christian church had become totally autocratic and power crazy. It outlawed any healing outside of its organization and executed all lay healers who dared violate its rules. Eventually, it was decreed that anyone who disobeyed its edicts would be executed on the theory that whoever disobeyed an ordained minister disobeyed God himself.

By that time, the European world was linear and strict. Ecstatic experience of the Divine went out the door. Much like today, fear was everywhere. God was not to be experienced directly, but only through appointed representatives—members of the clergy. Esoteric information about healing was hidden in books that only priests and the elite were allowed to read.

Most of this knowledge was lost to the general population, but saved by special, underground sects. The Christians had the Templars and remote monasteries; the Jews had the Kabbalah; and in the Islamic world, the Sufis carried the mystical secrets. In the East, esoteric secrets were kept alive with somewhat more visibility, mainly because of the guru system in India and the monastic system in China and Tibet.

Humanity went from a belief in gods that held the properties of both light and dark, good and evil—since those earlier generations had understood the unity principle that All Is One—to a belief in a single god who held only goodness and light. (Today we perceive the God of the Old Testament as vengeful, but His actions were viewed as appropriate in the context of the times; therefore, He, too, was revered as a God of light.) That meant we needed to project the darkness onto something else, which became women and nature, where it still remains. When ordinary people sought relief from this narrow view and began to worship the Virgin Mary, church authorities allowed it so they wouldn't have a complete revolt on their hands.

As ancient civilizations were conquered—Egyptian, Chinese, Greek, and Roman, among others—all of the libraries that housed the esoteric wisdom of their civilizations, including how to effect healing, were burned. The period that followed, the early Middle and Dark Ages, was a time when the mysteries were lost to all but a select few, and science and religion were in diametrically opposite camps.

The Middle Ages of the 11th, 12th, and 13th centuries also gave rise to the Inquisitions and the Crusades. The Inquisitions were necessitated by the fact that the populace was becoming better educated and more restive under the strict rule of the Catholic Church. The totalitarian regimes could pull people from their homes in the middle of the night, force them to endure humiliation, and then publicly execute them later on. This kept everyone in line, especially anyone using midwifery or herbs, both of which were completely prohibited.

However, the mysteries were protected, hidden from view, and preserved and passed down from masters to initiates by secret societies—groups I've found in every culture I've visited or studied. In many places, rituals and practices were kept alive through oral tradition, as with the Native Americans. A great deal of ancient knowledge was also preserved in the Vedas of the East Indians; as a result, India has always had talented healers and teachers.

By the time the Western church went to war during the Crusades, it was essentially waged against anyone who was not Christian, especially Muslims and Jews. One Crusade completely eradicated an entire group in France that practiced a combination of Christianity, Sufism, Kabbalah, and nature worship because they allowed women to be priests.

As Europe entered the age when the printing press made reading and writing much more available, the Protestant Reformation in the early 1500s broke the thousand-year rule of the Catholic Church. The good news was that it shifted the power base from priest to layman. Unfortunately, though, Martin Luther, John Calvin, and their colleagues held an even more austere view of human life than those they rebelled against, further obliterating healers and their rituals, balms, and practices. And while Luther and Calvin both honored Mother Mary for her faith and role as the mother of Jesus, they completely disapproved of those Marians who would elevate her to the same divinity as Jesus. The entire role of women in general, and female healers in particular, was pushed even farther off the world stage.

The Divine Feminine

In reviewing history, we see that as the dark side of human consciousness—and it's crucial to understand that we all have one—was buried deep in the personal and collective unconscious, so was the Divine Feminine. Female deities and goddesses were erased from memory, their statues and holy places destroyed or built over. Prayers to them became grounds for execution. The entire Divine-Feminine archetype was sent underground. The human body itself, as I've noted, was declared to be sinful, and women themselves were the fount of all evil. Everything about the body became forbidden: pleasure, passion, sensuality, and sexuality. Even dancing, laughing, and having fun were considered immoral. Women, especially healers, didn't stand a chance.

When the persecution of witches got under way, thousands of women and quite a few men were burned at the stake for practicing some of the very techniques that I teach today. Women who refused to confess their heinous crimes and recant their ways suffered horribly. Everything that was magical, mystical, or connected to nature was driven far below the surface of everyday life. The Divine Feminine didn't resurface into general thought again until Carl Jung's concept of the collective unconscious opened the door to the rediscovery of the feminine principle and healing in modern times.

Contrary to popular belief then and now, the body and the soul are not separate, and the body itself is not evil. It has never been less Divine than the soul. The reemergence of this awareness is at the core of the current wave of interest in the goddess and the feminine face of God, the Sacred Feminine. And it is in this awakening environment that energy medicine is once again taking its rightful place.

19th-Century Healing

Mysteries were last publicly seen in the West in the rituals of the ancient Greek Mystery Schools at Delphi and the practices of the early Christian mystics. Then they seem to disappear from view for centuries, as did women healers after the witch hunts. But both resurfaced with the early British Theosophists, a group that practiced religious philosophy and mysticism, in the 1800s.

Alice Bailey

The most famous Theosophist was Alice Bailey (1880–1949), and though not a healer herself, she was an influential writer and thinker. Her inspired words and teachings on spirituality cover a host of topics, including astrology, meditation, healing, Christianity, the occult, and even politics. Alice visualized a world where there was only one society with one global religion linked to the Age of Aquarius, that part of the vast cycle of astrological ages we are currently ushering in.

She claimed that the majority of her work was telepathically dictated to her by an inner-plane Tibetan monk named Djwhal Khul, and I don't doubt it. Her religious writings would be considered heretical by any church; in reality, they are probably much closer to the beliefs of the original followers of Jesus, dating back to the first 75 years after his death.

Recently, Alice was criticized for purportedly racist and anti-religious writing, but if you read her I think you'll find that her work is easily misunderstood because her thinking was just so outside of the box.

Mary Baker Eddy

One of the first people to attempt to re-create the healing power of the Christ light, Mary Baker Eddy is frequently described as the most influential female figure in modern religious history. In the mid-1800s, when this New Englander was in her 30s and 40s, she was fascinated by the possibility of instantaneous healing. She studied homeopathy and mesmerism (the forerunner to hypnotism), but those systems didn't exactly click for her. Neither did marriage—she divorced her cheating husband and had to take handouts from her better-off relatives.

Mrs. Eddy had been in ill health much of her life when she slipped and fell on some ice at age 45, causing a severe spinal injury. Her neighbors carried her into the nearest home, where the doctor told her to prepare for death. As was common practice for the society she lived in, Mrs. Eddy was a devout Protestant, so she asked for her Bible and readied herself to die. While reading about one of the miracles performed by Jesus, she suddenly had a spontaneous healing, got up from her deathbed, and went downstairs for dinner.

Soon Mrs. Eddy began to accomplish very impressive healings on others, and she trained her followers to do the same. The local churches rejected her, so she started her own group, calling them Christian Scientists. A religion with a strong presence to this day, its followers are not actually considered Christian because they believe that Jesus was a highly enlightened human being, but not God.

I've worked closely with Mrs. Eddy's followers, and they are very well-educated, thoughtful people who strive to live much like the early Christians did. They spend a fair amount of time every day in prayer and study, place little emphasis on material possessions, don't drink or smoke, and tend to live well into their 90s and 100s. They believe in self-healing, but don't impose their beliefs on others; they are remarkably open-minded and don't judge other ways of life.

Mary Baker Eddy wrote her classic book, *Science and Health*, in 1875. It has sold over ten million copies, and is still a best-seller today. She dedicated her life "to commemorate the word and works of our Master, which should reinstate primitive Christianity and its lost element of healing."

I spent years studying Mary Baker Eddy and her work, trying to decipher the secret she had stumbled upon as she lay dying that cold winter evening. I've concluded that she figured out how to emulate the healing power of Jesus and reproduce that same effect. My theory is that she learned how to re-create a force field of unconditional love, which requires a fully open heart chakra.

Mary Baker Eddy lived to be 89, speaking and writing and healing right up to the day of her death. Her followers did their best to continue her work, but after just a few decades, they'd lost the healing touch . . . just as the followers of Jesus had.

20th-Century Healing

When I really started looking intently for people throughout history who had mastered healing, I searched high and low, East and West. The few I found are those listed in this chapter. Most noteworthy are three women: Mary Baker Eddy, whom we've just discussed, and the two coming up next: Agnes Sanford and Kathryn Kuhlman.

Agnes Sanford

Agnes Sanford was born in the late 1800s to Presbyterian missionaries living in China. She married an Episcopalian priest and dutifully tried to be a quiet and unassuming wife, but failed miserably on that score. Like Mary Baker Eddy, Agnes had her share of marital problems, as her husband was inclined to be jealous of her mystical abilities.

And she certainly did have a knack for healing. Similar to Mrs. Eddy, she could simply focus on people who were sick and the next thing they knew, they were well. She wrote a book called *The Healing Light,* which I learned a great deal from, but it didn't become quite as famous as Mrs. Eddy's. In it, she describes the healer's attitude as one of "perfect open-mindedness," and relates the following about her practice of healing: "The first step in seeking to produce results by any power is to contact that power. . . . The second step is to turn it on. . . . The third step is to believe that this power is coming into use and to accept it by faith." Finally, she says, "No matter how much we ask for something it becomes ours only as we accept it and give thanks for it."

Agnes said that love was the most powerful healing force in the world—did she have that same incredibly open heart chakra that Jesus did? Agnes continued to perform healings until she died a peaceful death, and her work pretty much died with her.

Kathryn Kuhlman

By far the most colorful of the lot, Kathryn Kuhlman was born in the early 1900s. She was an itinerant preacher during the Great Depression, and after she'd been on the road for many years, during which she preached in a different town every night, miracles started to occur during her services. Once Kathryn became famous, she began appearing in larger venues. To silence detractors, she'd have a panel of Jewish rabbis, Catholic priests, and physicians from Harvard sit on the stage with her and attest to the authenticity of her work.

Kathryn also had her problems with the opposite sex. (This does seem to be a universal theme with these women healers!) She fell in love with a married man, and he divorced his wife to be with her. This blew apart her ministry, and it eventually forced her to leave him in order to continue her work. Of course, that kind of sacrifice only made her miracles all the more powerful.

I've read Kathryn's meager writings and watched DVDs of her work, and there is no doubt that she put herself into "the zone" through prayer. Once there—in an altered and expanded state—healings started to occur in the audiences sitting in front of her. It's very impressive to watch, although, like so many of the religious healers I've personally studied with, Kathryn wasn't able to direct these powers to specific individuals.

From my research on this extraordinary woman and her work, I concluded that she had opened her heart chakra to such an extent that she, too, was in some sort of advanced state of unconditional love. In fact, I studied all three of these women—Mary Baker Eddy, Agnes Sanford, and Kathryn Kuhlman—in great detail. It is my belief that they had each managed to merge with the energy field of the master healer, Jesus, whom they followed. They simply aimed to do the work of their mentor and guide. He is the one who figured it out, and somehow they managed to reproduce his work—if only during their lifetimes. All three were able to perform instantaneous healings; although, as I mentioned, Kathryn Kuhlman wasn't able to focus hers on specific individuals. The other two women were able to look you in the eye and say, "You're next. You will be healed," which is another incredibly impressive spiritual step up.

Other Pioneers in Energy Medicine

Energy medicine owes a debt to several other pioneers whose efforts have greatly increased our understanding of the energy field and the mechanics of healing the human body.

— **Dr. John Pierrakos** began his groundbreaking work in the United States in the 1950s. He was a big fan of psychiatrist Wilhelm Reich, and the two talked of an energy field they called *orgone,* which we now call the unified field. John then joined forces with another student of Reich's, Alexander Lowen, who was a controversial psychiatrist. Together, the two developed a study they called *bioenergetics* that allows practitioners to analyze the inner lives of their clients.

— John's wife, **Eva Pierrakos,** was a medium and trance channel who developed a spiritual system she called *Pathwork.* Over the course of 30 years, she gave 258 lectures that laid out the foundation for a journey of personal transformation and wholeness. John's association with Eva deeply affected him, and his work started to take on a spiritual component that he called *psychodynamics.* They weren't healers per se, but together they moved modern healing concepts forward.

— In the 1970s, **Valerie V. Hunt,** the Professor Emeritus of physiological science at the University of California, Los Angeles (UCLA), received a grant to study the effects of structural integration, or *Rolfing,* a therapy that had both physical and emotional healing components. In the course of her research, she conducted an experiment that measured the electrophysical activity of the human body while the color frequencies in the subject's energy field were viewed clairvoyantly from another room.

— Working hand in hand with Dr. Hunt was **Rosalyn L. Bruyere**, the clairvoyant who was vital in actively establishing hands-on healing here in the U.S. Their experiments led Dr. Hunt to conclude that what science called the human energy field was precisely what Eastern systems were referring to when they spoke of the aura, or the "auric field," which were generated by the energy vortices known as chakras. Thus did East meet West at UCLA.

— **Barbara Brennan** picked up the mantle from Rosalyn back in the '60s and began teaching hands-on healing to her students; she is largely responsible for the reemergence of energy healing in the West in recent times. Barbara was a respected scientist at NASA before moving into the healing field, thus bringing quite a bit of credibility to it. I graduated from an energy-healing school—the Mystery School I mentioned earlier in the book—that taught many of the same concepts as the school Barbara Brennan founded, and then went on to teach that work. I had spent many years prior to that doing similar work under the auspices of various esoteric religious groups and with South American shamans.

During the years I spent in the intensive study of healing, I worked within two distinct frameworks: what I call the Christian camp and the New Age camp. The similarities between them are far more significant than the differences—both seek connection with Divine energy with the intent to heal—and yet rarely do these groups overlap with each other. The New Age types largely shun traditional Western religion, while those who practice healing within a religious context consider their approach the "right way" and may fear and disparage New Age teachings as "occult."

What I usually found as I moved back and forth between the two sides was that the New Age groups had great techniques but not much connection to Source, and the Christians often had a great connection to Source but poor techniques. For instance, they didn't have any concept about how to protect themselves from psychic attack. (We will discuss this at length later in the book.) The South Americans were an interesting combination of some elements of each camp, while they also incorporated aspects of their unique indigenous roots.

New Age systems, like those of their Christian counterparts, are more accurately described as *esoteric,* insofar as they focus on what is unseen or hidden to the objective, fact-seeking mind. But healing is quintessentially nondenominational. This force of the universe cares little for our treasured yet limited beliefs, except as they support our development along the healing pathway.

21st-Century Healing

According to astrologers, we are in the beginning of the Age of Aquarius, or the age of the common man and woman. In the ancient world, it was believed that this would be the time when all of the lost mysteries would be revealed to ordinary folks, as opposed to being held solely by members of the clergy or intelligentsia. I believe that this time has indeed come. We see it happening with increasing regularity: in new physics, new biology, and a new approach to medicine. We now have the choice to pick up the mantle and carry the ancient knowledge into the future.

Are *you* going to be among those who carry the mystery of healing forward?

EXERCISE: Your Healing Lineage

Before we move on to the next chapter, where you will have the chance to examine your beliefs, take some time to think about the healing modalities you are presently most comfortable with. Do you maintain your health with regular visits to an acupuncturist and get relief from symptoms with Chinese herbal cures? What about Tibetan medicine? Do you go strictly to board-certified medical doctors? Do you trust male practitioners more than female ones? Do you have experience with a wide range of alternative treatments, such as homeopathy; flower remedies; or hands-on healing from chiropractors, naturopaths, osteopaths, or energy healers? Have you ever had a tribal shaman—from any Native American lineage—do a healing ceremony with you? Are there any traditions or specific cultures that make you uneasy?

Also, spend some time thinking about your lineage. Do you have ancestors from some part of the world who practiced a particular healing tradition? Are there any hints that there was a witch burned to death in your family tree? What about an itinerant preacher who was known to lay on hands? Or a grandmother who read auras? Midwives? Herbalists?

Take some time to write in your journal about any of these questions, or any concerns that they might have raised about your personal approach to healing.

It's an interesting exercise to connect to your roots and perhaps discover a hidden mystical thread in your history. Ask yourself what you believe . . . just in time to shake it all up in the next chapter.

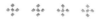

chapter four

EXAMINING
YOUR BELIEFS

In order to study healing around the world, from ancient to modern times, and be able to learn techniques from various cultures and the historical relevance of different traditions, I had to completely open myself to all systems of thought—especially those that appeared to be in total opposition to my own. When I started that process, I'd just had a mind-blowing recovery from cancer. I use the term *mind-blowing* intentionally because that's what it felt like: as if my mind had been blown open and I could think clearly for the first time.

Having experienced a remission at the hands of an energy healer, my first inclination was to understand the techniques that this person had used on me and go full bore into working with the chakra system. But Spirit, with its great sense of humor, decided to take me in a different direction.

How I Learned to Examine My Own Beliefs

I was coming out of a hospital—where I'd had my very last frightening and invasive test to confirm that I was indeed disease free—when I stumbled into a kiosk that had flyers in it about healing. Curious, I took one back to my hotel and read fascinating stories about real people who'd had instantaneous healings using something that sounded suspiciously like prayer. I consciously put aside my extreme antireligious feelings of that time, called the number on the flyer, and attended the next meeting of what turned out to be a mystical Christian healing group. I was intrigued by the group's work, and began to study with its members in earnest. In order to do so, I had to rethink the strong sentiments I'd had against religion ever since I'd walked away from Catholicism at the age of 15, swearing I'd never set foot in a Christian church again.

I actually ended up spending many years learning from these healers, who truly practiced what they preached. They taught me so much about the need to examine my own beliefs, which was an exercise they themselves did on a regular basis, calling it *discernment*. No matter how crazy of an idea I came up with, they never shot me down, but instead said, "Let's use our discernment to examine that belief." They were absolutely the most open-minded folks I'd ever been around, and they had some amazing abilities when it came to healing through prayer.

While studying with this group, I realized that I had been so busy between the ages of 15 and 25 rejecting the spirituality of my childhood that I'd also accidentally dismissed what I'd learned about miraculous healings. As I was renouncing Catholicism, I'd thrown out Christianity at the same time—I'd been so vehemently opposed to these organized religions. Like so many others in my age group, I was perfectly comfortable with Eastern devotions such as Buddhism and Hinduism, but not with anything Christian or Jewish. I was certain that there was nothing of value in the Western faiths, so I had to completely revise my thinking when I started out in the healing field.

I ultimately left these wonderfully gifted people because I wanted to study hands-on healing, which was a specialty they did not offer. But I can't thank them enough for all they taught me about their techniques and the need to be receptive to new ideas.

I later enrolled in the Mystery School I talked about before, which focused on the chakras and energy, or hands-on, healing.

I'd only been there a few days when the head teacher demanded to know where I'd learned to do such effective "distance healing," which my earlier training would have called prayer. Being naïve, I volunteered that I'd been taught that technique in a Christian setting. Upon hearing this, she promptly closed her mind and blocked any further discussion of the topic. She obviously had a limiting belief from her childhood that all organized religion was negative. No way could she accept the fact that a group like that might have something of benefit for her. Years later, when I was an instructor of energy healing myself, and I co-taught with that same individual, she confided that she had been sent home at the age of 12 by her Baptist choir director for wearing a skirt he deemed too short. At that very moment, she'd thrown all religion out the door, the baby along with the bathwater, never to reconsider it again.

One thing I figured out from that early experience in Mystery School was to keep my mouth shut about any skills I'd acquired over in the Christian camp. And while that esoteric group of healers I'd worked with had been broad-minded and educated to the extreme, I can assure you that I went on to study with numerous other Christian healers who were just as fearful of others' methods as my Mystery School teacher had been.

I remember one preacher in particular who told me that I'd been exposed to evil spirits and needed an exorcism because I'd spent time inside Hindu temples when I was in India and Nepal. But that same person had an amazing technique of bringing down the Holy Spirit to his followers, and I learned something from him, too. If I'd slammed shut my mind when he'd been so negative with me, I wouldn't have had the opportunity to learn what he had to offer.

The Power of Unconscious Beliefs

Why is it so important to routinely examine your beliefs? Because some of them may be limiting you, may be holding you back—especially those that stem from fear-based thinking. Fear is always limiting, as opposed to expanding. When you start to look closely at your particular beliefs, you may be surprised to find that some that are entrenched actually close doors rather than open them.

When I was trying to get to the root of my cancer, I really dug into the content of my thoughts and was surprised to find that I held many that were very limiting. I spent years coming up with a pretty comprehensive list of all my beliefs, examining each one carefully and then making a conscious choice whether or not to keep it. If I decided that a certain mind-set no longer served me, I intentionally discarded it and replaced it with a new one that I'd given serious consideration based on rational thought. To this day, I still check my thinking regularly. Every time I am exposed to something that I disagree with (like the death penalty), I still go through the same exercise of identifying and examining my underlying feelings that run counter to what is presented.

Often, our most important beliefs are unconscious. Over 90 percent of those that we currently hold we took on as kids from our parents or caregivers, school, and culture. These views run the greater part of our lives and determine if we're going to be happy or unhappy, rich or poor, healthy or unhealthy, and broad-minded or narrow-minded on different topics. If we stop to think about this for a moment, it's positively frightening. We inherit what we believe, most of which is unconscious, and all of it dramatically influences our lives!

For instance, you may know a little bit about John of God, the renowned spiritual healer of Brazil. You likely assume that he practices some form of indigenous healing, since his center is way out in a remote area of Brazil. Chances are, you've already decided that he's okay in your belief system. Well, I've worked with John of God, and he's actually quite religious—an interesting mix of Catholicism, Spiritism, and a little magic from Africa thrown in for good measure.

Many of the rituals at his center are quite Catholic in nature. Yet there are people who come from all over the world, from all faiths, to seek his help. I found being there a highly charged spiritual experience . . . think about what I would have missed if I had put up my old antireligion block.

Do You Actually Know What You Believe?

Questioning your beliefs is an exercise well worth engaging in. It will free you from all kinds of limitations in life, including fear and living according to what's right for someone else but not for you.

You'll want to ask yourself: "Where did this belief come from?" and "Does it still work for me, or is it limiting me in any way?" If you think that an idea no longer fits or is hampering you in some way, ask yourself what might suit you better at this time. Trust me, you *can* change your beliefs. I've done it countless times.

Here are some of the major areas you'll want to check:

— Let's start with **your religion,** since it's always the primary limitation for people when they want to expand their consciousness. What, if any, childhood faith were you raised in? Do you believe in the tenets of that faith now? Do you practice them? Are you aware of unconscious beliefs from your early education about religion that may be negatively affecting your life today?

When I was in my teens and early 20s and went through my very antireligious period, part of my rejection of my Catholic upbringing had to do with distancing myself from everything my family believed in. For example, I wanted to go to a liberal-arts college on the East Coast, but my mother would only pay for my tuition if I went to a West Coast Jesuit university so she could continue to keep me under her thumb. I acquiesced grudgingly, but with blinders on. Unfortunately, I refused to take in what those brilliant and highly educated teachers had to offer. I even challenged their standard requirement of taking two years of theology. They, being broad-minded, agreeably waived it for me, and it was a decision I later regretted. Imagine how much I could have learned from the Jesuits about such an important topic.

— Consider your beliefs about **the religions of others.** Do you automatically reject others or their thinking because their religion is different from yours, even if you, at best, give only lip service to your own? For example, I have a friend who refuses to become involved in any activity that utilizes Christian principles because he was turned off to these organizations as a child by exposure to proselytizing evangelicals. As a result, he missed out on the great time I had with this group, learning to speak in tongues and the techniques they use to effect some pretty amazing spiritual transformations.

— Then there's the elephant (and the donkey) in the living room—**politics.** So many people automatically exclude everything from the "other side," assuming that no good can come from it. For example, I have several liberal friends who refuse to watch Fox News. Yet this network has had me on numerous times to talk about a host of different subjects—from why young girls shouldn't get breast implants to why prescription-drug abuse is such a problem today.

Do you automatically decide that everyone who opposes your viewpoint is 100 percent wrong? How much do you expose yourself to the beliefs of the other camp? Do you listen exclusively to NPR and read only The Huffington Post? Or do you only get your news from Glenn Beck? To broaden your thinking, read from and watch media outlets that aren't in complete agreement with your belief system.

— What about your **social values?** For example, where do you stand on abortion, the death penalty, gay marriage, and other important topics? I always try to read well-written pieces on both sides of every issue and then consciously recheck my position. Have you thought through your own views on these issues recently, or do you automatically determine that there can be nothing of merit in the other argument?

— How about your beliefs about **race?** We'd all like to think that we're blind to skin color, but the truth is that we inherit racial prejudices from our family of origin, our schools, and our country —and these are very hard to delete. Many of us who live in the southwestern part of the U.S., for instance, are inclined to assume that if an individual looks Hispanic, he or she is likely to be an illegal immigrant.

Or how about your feelings about those people on the plane who appear to be Middle Eastern and are automatically pegged as terrorists . . . but it turns out they're Jewish and live only a few blocks from you?

— Then there's **gender,** my personal favorite. When I was a young attorney entering the appellate court to argue my first case, the clerk, herself a woman, assumed that I was a secretary. Our stereotypes about gender have improved over the past 25 years, but we still have a long way to go.

How often are you surprised when a doctor turns out to be a woman instead of the man you were expecting; or, even more surprising, an African American or East Indian woman? Turning again to my own life, I was taken aback recently when my bank suddenly made my husband the primary holder on an account I'd had in my own name for years. The employee who made the automatic judgment call that the man of the house should be the main account holder was, as you might suspect, a woman.

— How about **class differences?** That's such a sticky subject that people are afraid to even bring it up. What goes through your mind when you see someone who's dressed like a bag lady? If there's one thing I learned as an attorney, it was to never judge a book by its cover; frankly, many of my most affluent clients looked as though they were living on the streets. Or, conversely, do you assume that all trust-fund babies are spoiled brats?

— Don't forget your beliefs about **money.** I can almost guarantee that if you have money problems, they can be traced back to certain beliefs you inherited from your family of origin.

— And you can't forget about **relationships.** It's a fact that you are much more likely to stay married if your parents' marriage held together. What subliminal or overt messages did your mother and father give you about relationships?

— What about **weight?** If you're too heavy, how negative are you with your self-talk? Are your extra pounds what you hate most about yourself? How much time do you spend worrying about your weight as opposed to thinking about the time you could devote to helping others—a far better way of judging yourself?

— Then there's **food.** Do you believe that some foods and certain diets are good, while others are bad—that being a vegetarian or vegan or raw-food advocate is almost sacred and the only way to go? When I studied with a group of healers who convinced me of the importance of eating meat, I had to do a complete 180-degree turn, as I'd been a vegetarian when I arrived at their center.

Why Is It So Vital to Question Your Beliefs?

Most of your preconceived beliefs are unconscious unless you make the effort to shift them into your awareness. I'm urging you to bring all of them to your consciousness for a number of important reasons:

1. Your unconscious beliefs may inhibit you from becoming all that you are meant to be. It's nearly impossible to expand and grow, to take in new information and make new choices, when you are confined to operating solely according to preexisting ideas. Part of your task in life is to reach beyond the bounds of your conditioning and live true to who you want to be. You can't do this if you don't question your unconscious beliefs.

2. If you want to learn to work with others, you'll need to be able to accept their beliefs and treat them with the same respect you would your own. You will find this hard to do if you've got a fixed mind-set. Aspiring healers often want to shove their ideas about health or food or exercise or whatever else down their clients' throats. But that isn't healing; in fact, it completely blocks the healing energy. Take, for example, the insistence that someone quit smoking (based on the belief that smoking is always bad). A better solution is to be open-minded to the possibility that this person might need this habit until he has more recovery time

under his belt from a far more serious addiction to prescription drugs.

3. A person with a lot of fixed beliefs is acting from fear. Being afraid to give serious thought to the activities and opinions of others means that you are judging them without really giving their ideas your full consideration.

From an energetic perspective, closing yourself off to anything requires you to shut down your energy field to some extent. Alternatively, you want to be open to every idea, every practice, unless and until you have thoughtfully—"prayfully," as the esoteric Christians would say—determined that it is counter to your well-being or your ethics to such an extent that you cannot entertain it.

By taking you through the way one of my beliefs was fortunately amended, I'll hopefully be able to demonstrate how limiting beliefs can stifle your potential as a healer, and how those beliefs can be changed.

After working in the hands-on-healing arena for many years, and never seeing anyone throw down his or her crutches and walk, I'd absorbed the subliminal belief that real physical healings rarely happen. Maybe they did at Lourdes, the French village where so many miracles have occurred, or in the presence of a healer such as Kathryn Kuhlman, who was described as "the one-woman Lourdes," but certainly not around an average wannabe like me. I had taken on the idea that complete healing is rare and not to be expected. If one should manifest, I assumed it would only happen gradually, over time. After all, I'd learned that the physical body takes a while to reflect the changes that have occurred in its energy field. Instantaneous results are not commonly seen, and we shouldn't anticipate them. That was what I had been taught by the Mystery School teachers, and it was a belief I had fully employed.

One day after a meditation, I suddenly wondered: *What would shift this paradigm?* Knowing how pervasively our expectations govern what can and cannot occur, I began to work on the subtle level of my own thoughts to shift my presumption and allow for the possibility of instantaneous healing. Something deep in my bones told me that this was the most important aspect of my work: to think outside the box and allow for the *possibility* of miraculous healing—not just for me, but for others as well.

While I strived to improve my healing ability, I also continued to practice other skills. Mystery School had taught me many useful techniques, which I incorporated into what I'd acquired previously with the Christian healers. I learned to "drop into" the energy field and body of another person (to literally move my consciousness there) and hold focused awareness on a "key point," the place in his or her physical self and energy field that, if released, can open the floodgates of energy to support self-healing. I mastered the technique of calling in universal energy and directing it into someone's subtle field and body. In more advanced classes, I also gained the ability to move energetically through the brain. I even studied both subtle and gross anatomy and physiology, and an entire system of psychodynamics. Yet, up until that point, I hadn't actually healed anyone of a physical malady.

Working with a number of different teachers, I saw how an amazing transformation in the energy field of clients could occur. Some of those people even experienced slow physical improvement. But still, I never witnessed an instantaneous physical healing.

I looked into psychic surgery (which I will discuss later in the book) and healers such as John of God. While I loved working in his healing space, where more than 100 meditators help to hold the force field of energy, I didn't witness any miracles during my time there. I began to wonder if they could be achieved at all. Perhaps these wonders were only appropriate in the early days after Jesus, not to be experienced in *our* time. And yet, I had intensively studied the work of healers such as Kathryn Kuhlman and Agnes Sanford, both of whom performed healings as recently as the 1950s.

Then one day, a miracle happened right before my eyes. A woman I'd worked with a number of times on other issues called and said she had been in a car accident and had broken her wrist. When she came to my office, I examined her and could sense the break in the bone on both the level of her energy field and that of her body. Clairvoyantly, I also "saw" the fracture. I began directing focused intention to the area to increase blood flow and speed up her recovery. My expectation was that instead of taking the usual six to eight weeks to heal, it would mend in less time, maybe only four weeks. Suddenly, within the first five minutes of a one-hour session, I saw the bone heal. The break disappeared!

I gasped. I looked again to be sure I wasn't simply seeing the template of the bone in her energy field (where perfection always lies). Then I examined it once more. Her wrist was whole! I suggested that the woman have another x-ray. After she did, she called the next day to say that the break wasn't visible there either. I gave this incident quite a bit of thought in the ensuing weeks and months. Had I done anything differently that day? Could I repeat this phenomenon? I had no idea.

I returned to my practice with a new expectation of instantaneous healing. Still, clients came and went with no fanfare. Then, a young woman whom I'll call Jennifer made an appointment for a treatment at a healing school where I was teaching. She had a grade IV glioblastoma—the most aggressive form of brain cancer known. This 23-year-old wife and mother had little hope of recovery.

The lead teacher that day was working with Jennifer in the manner of this particular school, standing in front of the class beside a table where the patient lay quietly resting. I saw her shift her consciousness into the expanded, altered awareness that is often referred to as *healership*. In this state, the personality and "personhood" of the healer recedes as the Divine presence fills his or her body and mind. One of the most talented people I had worked with up to that point, she primarily brought through the healing presence of Isis. It always amazed me to see the shift when she would become this powerful Egyptian goddess before my eyes.

Not ten minutes into the treatment, the instructor looked up and began to scan the room with an intense, direct gaze that was unmistakably that of Isis. Zeroing in on me, she gestured and commanded: "Come here." This particular head teacher was a terror to work under, and I was sweating bullets as I walked to the front of the room. She then motioned to me and said, "You are to do this healing," and moved away from the table.

I stood beside Jennifer and held my hands, facing down, above her body, as is the standard practice in that environment. I began to scan and "read" her energy field as I'd been taught. Without warning, my hands changed their position, seemingly of their own accord, so that my palms were facing forward instead of down. I suddenly felt as if my heart broke—the pain was that intense. I was faint, and my heart enlarged a thousandfold and enveloped Jennifer. For a moment, everything became still. And that is when I sensed the presence of Jesus, the master healer, all around me. I saw his sacred heart on fire as he took my hands in his. I couldn't tell whose hands were whose, as ours intertwined as we ministered to Jennifer. The words I heard were: "From now on, you will heal this way."

At that moment, I had a strong knowing that Jennifer's heart had been healed, a step that was important for her peace of mind before she passed on. I also had a knowing that she would die soon. I was dumbfounded. I knew that I had been given a paradigm for instantaneous healing, but why hadn't this woman's cancer been healed? To this day, I am still examining my beliefs concerning healing versus curing, which we'll discuss in a subsequent chapter. For now, give some thought to the beliefs we've covered here and find out where you really stand. I think you'll find it to be a highly rewarding experience.

You'll find that looking clearly at your own beliefs is a lot like doing a major spring-cleaning. You toss out the clothes you haven't worn in five years, get rid of the chipped and cracked dishes in the cupboards, throw away the piles of paper that have magically accrued, and finally get around to vacuuming out the dust bunnies under the beds and in the corners of each room. When you've emptied out each garbage bag filled with your prejudices, doubts, and misguided ideas, and shaken out the dust rags of fixed beliefs, you can welcome in the fresh air of springtime that is now free to flow through your clean house. You are now ready to see what's been hidden under all of the chaos—the gifts of spirit that are your allies on the path to becoming your own shaman.

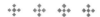

chapter five

BEYOND THE BASIC FIVE SENSES

Once you have examined your beliefs and opened yourself to new possibilities, and even briefly touched the unified field and tasted Oneness, certain abilities may begin to manifest. These expanded faculties have been termed *gifts of the spirit*, to use the language of religion, or *psychic abilities* as they are called in the secular world. They are sometimes a testament to, and manifestation of, Source working in and through you.[2] These gifts or skills are typically divided into three categories: *teaching gifts, sign gifts*, and *revelatory gifts*.

Teaching gifts are inspiring moments when someone is able to give understanding to another person or group on a specific point of difficulty or a challenge. It's as though the words are an actual infusion of light and clarity, delivered at exactly the right moment for maximum effect. We saw the beauty of this gift when Martin Luther King, Jr., gave his "I Have a Dream" speech. Delivered from the steps of the Lincoln Memorial, King's passionate words demanding racial justice and equality electrified America.

---

[2]It is possible to have tremendous paranormal powers and yet be coming from a place of darkness. Use your discernment and never give your power away simply because you're impressed by someone's psychic abilities.

His magnetism, sincerity, and emotion—all of which were clearly visible in his body and voice—infused listeners with a deeper recognition of the political and racial situation that was facing the country at that time. More than 40 years later, his words still ring with beauty and truth, awakening us to a vision of what peace could actually mean.

Sign gifts include the gifts of faith, healing, and miracles. They have the power to bring even the most skeptical individuals to their knees.

Finally, we have *revelatory gifts*, which include prophecy, the ability to sense beyond our reality, and speaking in (and interpreting) tongues. *Prophecy* here means when a person suddenly communicates with lucidity and authority, where the words are clearly coming from a source outside of him or her. Today, this would be termed *discernment* in the religious arena (not to be confused with the discernment of examining our beliefs), or *channeling* in the popular vernacular. We call abilities to sense beyond the norm *paranormal,* and that umbrella term includes feeling (clairsentience); seeing (clairvoyance); hearing (clairaudience); and touching, tasting, and smelling beyond the usual limits of those senses.

Speaking in tongues involves a spontaneous outpouring of seemingly unrelated sounds that has the energetic effect of connecting the communicator to Source. Often, one person will speak and another, likewise tapped into Spirit, will interpret the tongues. Many years ago, I visited dozens of random churches where I happily participated in this activity. "Tongues" can also be practiced alone as a very intimate form of prayer, often accompanied by a deep sense of joy and communion—it was said to be a favorite of Agnes Sanford. It's my sense that some indigenous people, with the help of dancing and drums, also speak in tongues when they are connecting to Spirit.

These gifts are always given for the benefit of the community, and not to boost an individual's ego. Once limited to ascetics and monks, today the gifts are available to all: students, housewives, working people—all manner of regular folks living otherwise ordinary lives, including you!

What Gifts Might You Already Have?

Every now and then, evidence of our innate paranormal abilities shows up in our day-to-day lives. Who hasn't heard of a mother who suddenly "just knew" that one of her children was in danger miles away? What about getting a phone call from the very person you were thinking about? Who among us hasn't sensed that we were about to get bad news, and then had our feelings confirmed? Even our military is said to use paranormal capacities as part of gathering intelligence, and the police and FBI have been known to call on psychics for help with certain investigations.

The information we usually get about the world around us comes through the normal five senses: sight, touch, taste, hearing, and smell. Our internal preferences and habits determine which sense, or combination of senses, we use in any given situation. Most of us get information primarily through images (visual) or sound (auditory); with touch (kinesthetic), taste (gustatory), and smell (olfactory) typically being the supportive modes to the two primary ones. Everyone is different, however—some of us even use different combinations at different times. It's heartening to know that in schools, more and more educators are becoming aware of different learning styles and trying to incorporate a variety of sensory approaches so their students have better access to the material being taught.

Another type of information that's available through these same sensory channels is *precognition,* or knowledge of a future event. Once you realize that every single fact—from the beginning of time through the present and into the limitless future—is available to you through the unified field, you will become open to receiving information about the future from any of the above channels.

Do bear in mind, though, that the future is malleable. It is possible to change and/or avoid certain events. That's because you have free will. For example, one time a client told me, "I can't wait to get my two teenage stepchildren out of the house." She complained that they were so much work and all she wanted to do was spend time with her husband, their father. As she spoke, I had a clear precognition that if she moved in the direction of urging the kids out of the nest, she would lose her husband. Despite my encouragement to focus on the children, she did indeed push them out the door . . . and when she called a year later for help, it was for support during a heartbreaking divorce.

When you first meet people, is your initial impression based on what they look like, the sound of their voice, or the feel of their handshake? Whichever sense is your strongest most of the time—and you do have a favorite—will be the one that you will find easiest to develop into a paranormal ability that you can have as a resource in your healer's toolbox.

As a healer, when you first meet a new client, you take in information about that person through all of your senses—the basic five plus whatever extended senses you are developing. What health problems is he facing? What is his biggest emotional issue? Where is the key point in his body or energy field right now that could turn everything around?

When I first started along the path of the shaman, I found that I could figure out what I needed to know about an individual simply by using my extended senses—essentially, I was using my own energy field and physical body to pick up what I could. This is not unusual for someone who has been traumatized. Trauma victims are often able to sense with their own bodies because they have developed a heightened sensitivity as a survival mechanism. Perhaps you were sexually abused as a child like I was, or have been physically or emotionally injured. Or maybe you were deeply afflicted by an illness or a surgery or an accident. It's possible that you became severely distressed as an adult while serving in the armed forces, in a situation of domestic violence, or while working for the boss from hell.

Our response to trauma makes us behave similarly to horses. Even though the domestication of this animal occurred many millennia ago, they spent much more time prior to that as prey. Their entire body and energy field evolved to be on the lookout for a predator. For those of us humans who have been treated as prey at some point in our lives, we are much more sensitive and able to pick up information at a distance than those who haven't, just as a horse does.

If any kind of trauma is part of your history, you will likely excel at developing your paranormal abilities and healing skills, since a rough life is often a prelude to receiving the gift of healing.

Mind vs. No Mind

When I was speaking at a conference not long ago, I met a woman named Sandy. She told me that she was 62 years old and had fallen twice in the previous year, breaking bones each time: a couple of ribs in the first fall and a hip in the second. The doctors told her that she had advanced osteoporosis and, naturally, she was quite worried. Sandy didn't have any idea what was causing such an advanced case at a relatively young age, so she'd come to me for help.

I began by asking her about her childhood, as I had a vague *knowing* that somehow it was related to her condition. At the same time, I *fell* into her energy field using my own body as a sensing mechanism. Sandy said that she was born with a hip deformity and had undergone several corrective surgeries before the age of two. This information dovetailed with what I got when she first walked up to me: a lot of fear and a disconnection from the natural world—that is, she didn't feel connected to the earth and she wasn't grounded. I concluded that this was likely the result of her early surgeries' damaging impact on her base chakra.

In Sandy's energy field, I sensed that her first chakra was distorted in shape and circling in the wrong direction, which means it was unable to take in energy and caused her to exhibit a distorted view of reality. She thought the nature of the world *was* trauma and pain and that there was danger lurking around every corner. She was also unable to receive any sustenance from Mother Earth, the source of all our strength and health. This explained the weakness of her bones.

Throughout this process, I went back and forth between "Mind" and "No Mind." We all know what the first term refers to: when we're thinking with our left brain. In my *Mind,* I was reviewing what I knew about the condition of osteoporosis and how it's often a result of a poorly functioning first chakra. From *No Mind*—that place in ourselves where we sense and feel, and from which we get our intuitions—I received information from the unified field and all of my senses, both normal and paranormal. This is how I obtained the information about Sandy's childhood and the fact that the base chakra's condition was a factor.

Next, I focused my attention directly on her physical body and found that her bones had that porous feel I associate with osteoporosis. Again, I moved between Mind and No Mind to arrive at this conclusion. At this point, I was pretty much done with the intake part of the session.

Working in an expanded state, I checked and deepened the connection with my guides (from years of doing this work, I am linked with them constantly). I specifically requested that they work through me, and then I expanded and raised my own energy field to accommodate their higher vibration. The guides began to resolidify Sandy's bones, using my body as the vehicle.

At the same time, I "heard" what Sandy needed to do in order to get well. Using that information, I gently explained to her that her bone problems were associated with those early childhood surgeries that had separated her from the earth. Therefore, reconnecting to it would help build bone health. I suggested that she walk barefoot on the beach (she lived very near the ocean) and spend time sitting with her back against a tree. These activities would put her in direct contact with earthly energies to further sustain bone strength.

When the guides had finished their work, I used my focused intention to firmly root Sandy's first chakra and sacrum directly into the earth. I did this without thinking; for me, it's as automatic as driving a car or brushing my teeth. I also recommended that she take up a practice like yoga, Pilates, or dance to bring her more fully into her body and aid in keeping the grounded connection I had helped her establish.

Some months later, I heard from Sandy. She reported that she was less anxious, more balanced, and peaceful. She had followed my suggestion and was taking dance classes. She had also formed the habits of eating outside at noon, sitting with her back against a tree, and walking barefoot in the sand at least three times a week. Her osteoporosis tests had improved dramatically, and she no longer needed to take medication for the condition.

Much of the information I received about Sandy, you would have picked up, too. In fact, you're probably already getting more than you realize about people's emotions and their health. When you become your own shaman, you will know how to go from getting occasional hunches to having fully developed intuitive skills. These are wonderful gifts of the spirit, and you will know that what you receive is highly accurate. Our culture calls advanced abilities "paranormal" or "beyond the norm," but that's only because 99 percent of modern humans have turned these sensing abilities off. The good news is that they can be turned back on rather easily.

Using Your No Mind

No matter the current condition of your No Mind abilities, they can greatly improve. They're probably just a little atrophied from lack of use; but like any muscle, they respond quickly once you start to exercise them. If you spend time in any of the creative arts—writing, painting, sculpting, or composing music—or if you meditate regularly, work with animals (especially horses), or spend time in nature in an expanded state, you will find it easy to develop your No Mind capacities.

The first, and usually the easiest, way to learn to sense another person through No Mind is by using what you feel in your own body. Some people pick up information from others most easily through their first, second, and third chakras; while for many, this is done through their fourth chakra. It is from your own chakras that you will most naturally pick up information about those you encounter, especially with regard to their emotions.

One time when I was a young girl, I took my dog to a training class. Afterward, the teacher had us all sit in a circle and "feel" into the different dogs. Each of us took a turn volunteering what we got from a dog we didn't know, and the instructor, who was privy to each dog's history, would verify our hunches or shoot us down. I happened to get a lot of answers correct, and the teacher told me, "You're reading these animals through your heart." I bet she was right.

When I was a lawyer, my partners would always tease me about my ability to predict what was going to happen in a case. I had no idea where I was getting the information, but I could be uncannily accurate about clients and the outcomes of their upcoming trials. Later, I realized that I was using what we call paranormal skills, but at the time it felt completely normal to me.

I also had a chance to be tested on getting information from others right after I had signed up for Mystery School. I showed up for the first lecture with yellow pad in hand, thinking I was going to be taking notes. Was I in for a surprise! One new student after another took the stage and answered a few questions, and our job in the audience was to identify their emotional states and related physical maladies, if any. I could tell which subjects were angry, which ones were sick and with what disorder, which ones were trying to recover from a divorce, and so on. The teacher told me I was getting a lot of my information through *clairsentience,* a French term meaning "clear sensing" that refers to our ability to feel others.

I believe that everyone is clairsentient to one degree or another. I'm sure you've walked into a room where you could sense the mood of the people in it. Or have you ever noticed how you can feel what the emotions were of the occupants of a home that has just been vacated?

As with most things, the best way to improve this skill is to practice. Every time you encounter someone, whether it be a family member, old friend, or new acquaintance, ask yourself what you're getting from him or her. Is that person happy, sad, or something in between? Does he or she seem hyper or relaxed? Intellectual or more earthy? Full of health or not? Those are some basic questions you probably consider already.

Then start to ask yourself more difficult questions. For example, if you'd had that brief meeting with Sandy, you might have wondered: *What is this woman's emotional state, and is it impacting her bones? Does her first chakra feel normal? Do her bones feel solid?* First hits are the best; they come straight from No Mind, which is almost always right, and not from Mind, which is so often wrong. You'll learn to be very quick with this process. If you have to ponder it, chances are you're in your Mind and guessing.

Here's an example of how information can come once you get a little more practiced at it. At a recent event where I asked for volunteers to join me on the stage, a man approached and, before he even spoke, I could sense that he had a broken heart from an old breakup. That information came to me using my own body and energy field (especially through my heart chakra) as a sensing mechanism. I also felt that his heart chakra was closed so that he could wall off the pain. Think of how many times *you* have picked up on someone's emotions and what his or her problems are before a word has been spoken.

For a moment, I saw in my mind's eye a quick flash of this man as a little boy and how abandoned he had felt at the time of his mother's death. That insight came through clairvoyance, which, as we'll discuss shortly, is connected to the sixth chakra. I also sensed that he had arteriosclerosis, hardening of the arteries, as a result of not dealing with the emotions of the old relationship (that information came from a direct sixth and seventh chakra knowing). This was something that he would have to have surgery for in the future unless he dealt with his blocked feelings (a precognition that came through the sixth and seventh chakras). Surprisingly, it only took a minute or two for all of that information to come barreling in.

Developing Your Clairvoyance

The sixth chakra, the third eye, is the center for visual, intuitive, and psychic perceptions—the ability to see beyond the limitations of time and space. Through this chakra, we can transcend our personal identity and gain entry to the universal field of all information—the unified field—where we can access guidance from beyond; telepathic communications; information regarding the future (precognition); information about remote locations (remote viewing); and visuals of images, scenes, and colors (clairvoyance).

Take a moment to imagine a coat in your closet. Picture its shape, its color, its buttons or zipper, and what's in the pockets. Even though it's in the closet and out of your line of sight, notice that you don't have any trouble seeing it. That means you have the ability to remember visually. Clairvoyance requires the same skill. You already have the basic equipment; it's just a matter of getting it to work in a more refined way. The most important step is to simply relax and let it happen. Let impressions come your way without caring what channel they're on. When your clairvoyance starts to work, you will find that the images often flash by so quickly that you can barely take them in; oftentimes, they are just flickerings of color, especially at first.

Maybe you can already see energy fields around people or things, or the details of chakras. Don't worry if you can't, though, as that same information can be accessed through other channels. One of the most talented individuals I know in this area is not at all clairvoyant; he relies instead on his strong clairsentient skills.

A warning about clairvoyance and other paranormal abilities in others: I want to reiterate here that you need to be careful not to give your power away to someone just because he or she impresses you with certain special abilities. The psychic world is full of people who use their gifts to boost their flagging egos; they employ their skills to make themselves look bigger and better so they can take your power away. Don't buy into that and become disempowered. Your own intuitions are, ultimately, the most valid ones.

In my early 20s, I had some serious accidents that I could have avoided if I'd honored my sixth-chakra information. One was a horrific near-death experience in white-water rapids that I'll describe a little later in the book. That time I had a precognition that trouble was just around the corner, but I ignored it.

This is why I think it's important to include a quick exercise here, which you can do to begin opening your third eye and enhancing all of the skills of the sixth chakra that are described in this chapter.

EXERCISE: Opening Your Third Eye

For this exercise, you'll want to be in a quiet place where you can direct your entire focus within. Sitting comfortably in a chair, relax and clear your mind. Now, intend to open your third eye. To support your intention, place your middle finger at the bridge of your nose and push up while breathing deeply. Imagine that you are opening the eyelid that is located exactly between your eyebrows. In your mind's eye, see this chakra opening, thereby enhancing your extrasensory (third-eye) capabilities.

Do this for about 60 seconds. The goal of the exercise is not to gain information, but rather to practice opening the third-eye chakra. As you develop this skill, you will begin to have experiences sensing beyond your five normal senses.

Once the sixth chakra is open and you are able to access information through it, the key to increasing your abilities is to relax and let information come to you. Don't hesitate to use your imagination to picture what you hope to see while you're learning. That's perfectly okay.

To Get There, Let Go

I didn't have much experience with advanced hearing, tasting, or smelling until I had been in the healing field for some time. Then one day, out of the blue, I suddenly began to hear, taste, and smell things that other people couldn't. Believe me, this can be a little unnerving at first! Initially, I noticed that I was hearing tones while I was working with clients and, after a while, figured out what they meant. Since I've studied music, I wasn't surprised to find that minor tones signified illness, while major ones signified health. Sometimes I'd also hear a word or phrase, at other times entire sentences. During the same period, I also developed an uncanny sense of smell, and today I can smell the rotting odor of sickness in a person from quite a distance. And then there's my sense of taste, which comes in handy when I "taste" a chemical or drug that someone has ingested.

As you expand your perceptual abilities, don't be disturbed if you begin to hear—in what may seem like the most normal circumstances—phrases or sentences in your head containing information that could be helpful to the person or situation you are contemplating.

If you want to begin developing your extrasensory capabilities on your own, simply intend to allow Spirit to work through you. The greatest obstacle is being small-minded or afraid. Over time, trust will grow as it becomes easier and easier to surrender your personal will to Divine will.

Another common block is the urge many people feel to be in control. The world we live in encourages the development of a strong self-identity. We like to "have it all together" so we can "take the ball and run with it" and always "come out on top." All of this leads to a false sense of self-sufficiency and strengthens the urge to be in command. Yielding is misinterpreted as giving up, but in reality it gives us access to a far greater power than the small, egoic self. Once an individual gets a glimpse of the vast resources that come flooding in when he or she lets go of the need to maintain control, the resulting freedom can lead to a highly exalted state.

EXERCISE: No Mind Awareness

We're all constantly receiving information from our environment, but much of it doesn't make it into our consciousness. People would be amazed to learn how much they missed in any given scene. For one thing, we're all on sensory overload, and each year that gets worse. If we absorbed that amount of light, sound, and vibration consciously, we'd simply blow out, so our psyche protects us. Another related problem is that, culturally, we rely too heavily on our mind. This misplaced emphasis has resulted in the loss of much of our natural ability to sense. When we learn to relax and shift into No Mind awareness, we start to receive and experience images, impressions, and sensations that we would otherwise have missed.

The following process outlines steps to focus your awareness:

1. First of all, *relax*. Take a few deep breaths and let go of the part of you that "tries," your perfectionist part. You'll want to allow the right brain—the receptive, feminine, and intuitive side of you—to be present.

2. Next, *open* yourself. Take a moment to feel the ground beneath your feet, which will help open your lower three chakras. Intend to open your vertical power current, the energetic cord that runs up through your spine. Then intend to open your heart and feel compassion. Now, relax your brow area, and intend to open your third eye. Feel your scalp relax and intend to open the crown chakra at the top of your head.

3. Next, *lift*. Using your intention, imagine an elevator going up inside you, lifting your awareness through your energy field and body

up toward your higher self above your head. Imagine that there is a column extending above your head, which makes it easier for the elevator to lift. Let the earth energy—pushing upward from the center of the earth—come through the minor chakras in the soles of your feet, through the legs, and then up through your first chakra at the base of your spine to help propel your awareness skyward.

4. Finally, *connect* by consciously and intentionally forming a triangle between your heart, your third eye, and the person or thing being observed. Still using your intention, expand that triangle by moving the point at the third eye up to include your higher self; picture it as the eighth chakra about three feet or so above your head. Now you're ready to observe that person, place, or thing and get information. Allow all of your senses and feelings to receive, and allow your inner ear to hear vibrational tones.

With practice, you will be able to hone your awareness and innate perceptive abilities, and more readily observe, listen, and receive.

Working with Animals to Expand Your Gifts

Working in a healing capacity with animals can be a wonderful way to get started expanding your gifts. A Facebook friend, Natalie, told me that the day her beloved dog died, a small, skinny cat walked up the street and came directly to her and her children, as if he knew they needed him. She said the name "George" popped into her head. That night, as the family members were still crying about the sudden death of their dear dog, George purred loudly and rubbed Natalie's face, clearly telling her that it would be okay. Their new pet made it so much easier for everyone to adjust to the loss of their old one. Animals always know what we need and how to help us—the least we can do is try to heal them when they need our assistance.

I've always had lots of pets. When I was a child we had Goldie, a cocker spaniel; a boxer named Teddy; and a whole series of cats. When I went off to college, I even tried to take my beagle puppy with me, but the dorm supervisor made me turn around and drive it back home. What was I thinking?! After I got married, I also had dogs. For example, there was Dolly, our black Lab who would squeeze herself into the smallest space in the car so she fit in with all of the climbing and camping gear. She would then reinflate herself when we reached the campground. And I always had cats, as many as eight at one time.

When I finally accepted the fact that I wasn't going to have children, I started to collect animals in earnest and lived close to them on a remote ranch in the Sierra Nevada Mountains. I began with llamas, which I bred. Llamas are amazing animals! They meditate every day, kneeling and facing the rising and setting sun. The mothers are so devoted to their young and do all of their training with gentle admonitions and little nips, never with anger or violence.

One day I was standing in a field, looking at a possible llama for purchase, when the owner's horse suddenly galloped up. I was so startled by such a large animal that I quickly climbed a nearby fence for safety; I'd never actually seen a horse up close before! Afterward, I couldn't get it out of my mind. A few days later, I asked a neighbor if I could ride hers; and the rest was history. I wound up taking a whole year off from my day job as an attorney to immerse myself in what I called "the university of the horse." Today, I still have my very first horse, named Influence. He is a flashy, black Dutch warmblood, just like the horse in *National Velvet*. He now lives right outside my kitchen window in well-deserved retired bliss.

Thanks to Influence, I learned to talk to animals and heal them. It began one day after I'd had him for about a month. I was riding through the desert chaparral when I heard him say, "It's too hot, and my back hurts." I was so surprised that I almost fell off. I jumped down and looked him in the eye and could see him laughing. He has quite a sense of humor! From that day on, I started listening very carefully and discovered that you can actually hear animals communicate if you simply quiet your mind and use your intention. Those are the same steps I take when I'm getting ready to do healing work with people: I form an intention to listen to them very deeply, way below the level of speech.

I wanted Influence to be familiar with all kinds of animals so he would be less likely to spook. My goal was to avoid a situation where I could easily violate the cardinal rule of always keeping the horse between myself and the ground. That was a great excuse to start a collection: I acquired a dairy calf, a billy goat, chickens, ducks, and a pig, as well as peacocks and ostriches. While I was adjusting Influence to every creature, including the herd of llamas he lived with, I was getting a pretty good education in how to talk to them. I took classes in using healing touch on animals, which is actually quite a solid foundation for doing the same practice on humans, since animals (especially horses) are much more sensitive to touch than people are.

The first step is learning to hear what the animals have to say. They will always tell you what their problem is if you just tune in and listen. The easiest sense to develop initially is usually in the area of your third and fourth chakras, as you can feel your pet through these areas. You can also receive a great deal of information through the minor chakras in the palms of your hands.

EXERCISE: Healing Your Pet

Feel free to practice this exercise on your pets even if they are not sick or injured. The healing touch will only increase the love you have for each other.

1. Sit quietly with your pet, with nothing competing for your attention like the TV or other people, and say, "I intend to open all of my chakras for the purpose of hearing what my dog [or cat or horse or hamster] has to tell me."

2. Simply touch your pet all over, listening carefully at the same time. You may hear words or phrases with advanced auditory sensing, or you may sense what your pet is feeling and thinking through your hands or any of your chakras, especially the third and fourth. Your heart chakra is especially good for communicating with them if you're an animal lover. The love between you and your pet will open the heart chakra and also begin the healing process for you in any human-relationship trauma you've experienced.

3. Whether or not you've figured out exactly what your pet is trying to reveal, you can still "talk" to them with touch. You'll always want to use a very gentle caress, and be sure to include the palms of your hands as you do so, as they contain important chakras. Keep in mind that animals, as I mentioned, are more responsive than humans are to touch. This is because they are less blocked than we are.

There are two important related points: First, when you pet an animal, it creates a hormone in your body that enhances your nurturing abilities—not only toward them, but also with people. You'll always want to discipline your pet gently using your voice, not your hands, so as to reinforce your role as their safe protector. Animals don't understand anger or violence in humans, and they immediately lose respect for you if you lose your temper. And never use your hands in anger with them or they will begin to recoil from your touch out of fear.

Second, just like with a person, when you make a conscious effort to communicate and heal your pet, it automatically heals you, too. As you open your chakras to heal
others—of any species—you become healed yourself. That
is the beauty of energy medicine.

What are the practices that assist us in opening up to the gifts
involved in healing? In the next chapter we'll talk about the main
ones that helped me become my own shaman, and that can help
you do the same.

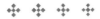

chapter six

WEAVING TOGETHER THE THREADS OF THE SHAMAN'S PATH

In addition to learning healing techniques, becoming your own shaman is dependent upon your clarity. Once you're clear within yourself, you can be a clear channel for others. How to get that clarity? The following five practices will be key to your development.

There's no particular linear order—as in, first do this, then that. Instead, it's more of a weaving together of various threads until you've become the whole cloth of an accomplished shaman. At the same time that you are clearing your energy field of blocks, examining your belief systems, and expanding your awareness in order to have a solid connection to the unified field and access to its powerful healing energy, you also need to be of service in some way so that you are giving to, as well as receiving from, the universe. Fortunately, these tasks are accomplished with fairly simple tools—surprisingly simple, in fact. A healer clears much of his or her own blocks and opens to receive ever-higher vibrations through the practices of journaling, meditation, prayer, forgiveness, and being of service.

Practice #1: Journaling

I'm sure you've heard the saying "The truth will set you free." But did you ever wonder why? Or how? If you've read my first book, *Truth Heals,* then you already have a fairly good idea.

Whenever life gets too difficult or threatening, such as when we experience an emotional or physical trauma of some kind—we may feel that we can't handle the truth and so we try to deny it. We send the facts about what is happening—and our resulting thoughts, beliefs, and emotions—underground, burying them deep inside us where we think we don't have to deal with them. We'll often distract ourselves with something less frightening, or even overwrite the truth with lies that, in the moment, feel safer—much like using the classic "I walked into a door" excuse to explain the bruises that actually came from domestic violence. We may lie to ourselves with things like "Oh, he really loves me," rather than consciously acknowledging the fear and danger that exist in a dysfunctional relationship.

The problem with this "Out of sight, out of mind," deny-and-dissociate strategy is that it doesn't work, at least not for long. Truth is a mighty force, a powerful energy that, like all others in our universe, exists in physical reality even if we can't see it with our eyes. Reality can't be wished away any more than gravity can. The truth exists, and it always will; this is a natural law of the universe. Therefore, dealing with it in a healthy way requires that it be processed. It needs to be moved out of the body and energy field—it needs to be released.

If this doesn't occur—if the truth about what happened to us and what we think and feel about it is not acknowledged, spoken, and liberated by the conscious mind—it will, like a beach ball that has been held underwater, eventually pop back up from the depths where it has been residing, giving rise to all sorts of attention-getting tactics. These issues that can resurface include emotional pain, abusive relationships, financial problems, accidents, health scares and conditions, and stress symptoms of all kinds—whatever needs to be done so that the truth can be dealt with and we can heal. Beneath almost any disturbance is truth waiting to be acknowledged and set free.

I first discovered this reality when I was dealing with cancer at age 25. As I've already discussed, it was the last in a series of wake-up calls I had been avoiding. Alcohol and prescription drug abuse, promiscuity, and extreme dieting had not been enough for me to realize that I had pent-up thoughts and emotions that needed to be healed. But the cancer was something I simply couldn't ignore . . . not if I wanted to live.

To my surprise, one of the simplest tools I found in my search for healing during that time turned out to be one of the most powerful. I discovered that writing in a personal journal gave voice (movement and release) to the truth about the traumas of my childhood. Journaling gave me the benefit of processing that old toxic energy that was stored inside me and had been wreaking such havoc on my life. Giving expression to the reality of my past ultimately led me to becoming cancer and addiction free, and to letting go of all the other lies I had been living.

We all have truths buried inside. Too often in childhood we are taught by our parents or society that feelings are bad and shouldn't be felt, let alone expressed. Stuffing down our emotions is the cultural norm. Yet in order to have a fulfilling life, complete with a healthy body and relationships, we have to own our emotions. They are a natural part of who we are. We need to experience them fully and then let them go. In essence, to truly be strong and joyful we have to live in truth. Journal writing helps us do that.

There aren't many rules to follow to gain these benefits. Here are a few guidelines for getting the most healing out of journaling:

1. **Do it daily.** Like brushing your teeth, create a habit that ensures good emotional hygiene. Get the old energy out, and then keep up the practice to prevent new toxins from accumulating.

2. **Use pencil and paper or keyboard and computer,** as both are equally effective. Your goal is a stream of consciousness, which will come about merely by using your body (your hands) to communicate.

3. **Be honest.** Practice rigorous honesty about your feelings no matter how petty, jealous, hateful, or anything else they may sound. It's time to honor your emotions, and this is the place to do it. Don't hold anything back.

4. **Don't edit, spell-check, or judge your writing.** That's not the exercise here. This isn't school, and you're not being graded. You're doing something far more important for your well-being, and that requires letting the thoughts and feelings flow uninterrupted.

5. **Keep your journal safe.** This means always placing it in a secure place where no one else will see it. To be uninhibited in your journal writing, you need to know that it won't be subject to the scrutiny of others.

6. **Share only if you want to.** If there is a trusted friend, therapist, or other loved one with whom you want to share your writing, by all means do so. Revealing your truth to another person, who then gives you unconditional acceptance, will increase your ability to process out the energy.

7. **Be committed to the truth.** Use your journal as a self-healing tool for your personal growth, self-improvement, emotional health, and physical well-being. Remember, the truth will set you free!

Daily journal writing will be a major step toward becoming your own shaman.

Practice #2: Meditation

Like journaling, meditation is crucial to our physical, emotional, and spiritual health. Every culture throughout history has had some form of meditation. The purpose of it is to still the mind; calm, cleanse, and refresh the body; and increase the connection to Spirit. If enough of us connect to Source and to each other, we will bring about a profound transformation of life on Earth.

As we've learned, thousands of years ago we could all see clairvoyantly, communicate telepathically, and easily feel into one another because we were all linked. We chose our leaders because of their wisdom, capacity to heal, and ability to tap into Source. We stopped using these skills over time, and it seemed that we had lost this knowledge. But it is not lost—it is stored in our DNA, in the very cells of our bodies. These abilities can be reactivated through daily practices of meditation and prayer.

Picture us all together again, living close to Mother Earth (and doing her no harm), intimately connected to one another and our Source. We can talk to the animals and feel the trees and the grass and the water as if they are part of our bodies. We talk to our ancestors and interact with one another through our thoughts. Each of us has a special talent, and we are respected for it and for the good it brings to all. Perhaps we excel at music, are good at working with herbs, or are natural leaders. And then there are those of us who can heal; we are shamans and priests, deeply connected to All That Is.

So how do you reclaim the gifts that are your birthright? One of the best ways is through meditation. The following is a basic exercise, called "the Microcosmic Orbit," which will lead you in that direction. It is easy and fun to do, and can be practiced every day, especially if you feel stressed or have trouble sleeping. It is an excellent practice to use in addition to meditation.

I highly recommend that you do learn to meditate, which, to be done correctly, requires studying with a teacher as opposed to picking it up from a book or CD. The exercises in these pages will serve as a good introduction until you have the opportunity to practice directly with an instructor. If you have a hard time finding one in your area, I teach it in my 21st Century Energy Medicine Program, both in person and via a live feed so you can learn from a distance. (For more information, see the Appendix.)

The Microcosmic Orbit practice is invaluable because it draws your attention to the flow of life force in your body. It is sometimes called the "warm current meditation" because of the way it directs energy, or chi. This famous practice dates way back to Taoist times in China, and its original principles can be found in the *I Ching*, which is more than 2,500 years old. The ancient Greeks, among other cultures, used this technique as well, calling it "serpent biting its own tail." You may have seen that symbol of the golden serpent biting its tail, which has been used to depict this particular process of transmutation.

Systems from two different cultures come together here in the sense that meridians (Chinese) in the body are pathways to the chakras (Hindu). Moving your energy along certain meridians will feed the chakras and can recycle, conserve, increase, and even transform the energy in your body and chakras into a higher form. Ultimately, this enables you to become aware of your higher self and assists in the development of your soul.

The Microcosmic Orbit can bring about extraordinary improvements in the quality of your life and health. It will give you a greater awareness and appreciation of consciousness and increase your resistance to illness and stress. However, if the food you eat is full of preservatives and additives, you may find that it's a bit slow going at first because the impurities in your body could be blocking your meridians. For faster results, eat and drink only foods and liquids that are fresh, additive free, and not full of sugar.

EXERCISE: The Microcosmic Orbit

For best results, practice the Microcosmic Orbit every day. It should take about five to ten minutes, so be sure to give yourself a quiet space and time when you will not be interrupted.

1. Sit in a comfortable position and take a deep breath. Set your intention to do the exercise and close your eyes. Let your tongue rest on the back of the roof of your mouth. If that's not comfortable, you can move it forward a little bit, but the farther back, the better.

2. Focus on your lower abdomen, about the width of three fingers below your navel and a third of the way into your body. Visualize or feel light, energy, and warmth accumulating in that location. Let them build there for a minute. Imagine, if you like, that you're blowing on the coals of a fire and they're glowing orange and becoming warm.

3. Now sense the warm energy flowing from that point toward your spine. To get there, it has to go down between your legs, over to your tailbone, and then up the spine. That's where the Microcosmic Orbit begins.

4. As you breathe in, imagine that the energy is going up your spine. Pause briefly when that warm energy goes up inside your skull and into the pineal gland at the center of your brain.

5. As you breathe out, see that energy starting to move down the front of your body. As it does so, feel that golden ball of warm energy going through the pituitary gland, which is just below the pineal gland and more toward the roof of your mouth. That energy is going to connect at the point that you have your tongue touching the roof of your mouth. From there it will go down your tongue and into your throat, as if you swallowed it.

6. Follow the energy down your throat and your esophagus, into your stomach, and then back down to the lower abdomen. Continue moving the energy into the bottom part of your torso, between your legs, and to the point just behind your genitals (the perineum). Then to complete the orbit, feel that energy go back over to your tailbone where it began.

In short, here's a summary of the route of the energy's orbit: As you breathe in, take the energy from the tailbone up to the pineal gland. Breathe out as you move it down the front of your body, between your legs, and back to the tailbone. Imagine with each pass that your vertical power current (the channel of energy that runs up your back in the location of your spine) is opening more widely.

This is the basic Microcosmic Orbit (which is a good prelude to developing a meditation practice). A more advanced form, which I teach in my 21st Century Energy Medicine Program, contains additional refinements that can help you clear your emotional baggage. (Again, for more information, please see the Appendix.)

The popular view of meditation is that its key purpose is to help us reduce stress, tune out, and get away from all the busyness and noise of daily life. Well, that's partially true. The real intention of meditation, though, is to tune *in,* to get in touch with what's inside of ourselves as well as with All That Is. The ultimate goal is to reach that state of peace within that so many traditions speak of—the kind that is beyond all understanding.

You may have heard of the discussion within quantum physics that there is a gap between your thoughts. Meditation is a way to get into that gap and extend it. It is in this space, this gap between thoughts, where you will find your entryway to infinite mind—that mystery some refer to as "Spirit" or "God." When you're in that space, that field, you'll find the true meaning of Oneness. You'll discover that you, everyone, and everything else are connected to each other and to All That Is. You'll also discover that this field is pure, boundless potential—that you can accomplish anything when you're tapped into it. You can create anything, heal anything. Meditation is the one intentional path that easily and reliably takes you there.

Meeting the Madonna

Now I'd like to share a story about how meditation prepared me for an amazing experience that helped me take a major spiritual step up.

I've spent a good part of my life studying the healings of Jesus and trying to understand and re-create them. While I certainly had my fair share of problems with the Catholic Church in my youth, one thing that this organization does well is implant a firm belief of miracles in its followers. As a child, I was certain I could make wonders happen for myself if I learned how to connect deeply enough with Jesus; his mother, Mary; and the other saints who performed them.

As I mentioned, I left the Church when I was in my teens—during my wild years of rebellion against all I had grown up with. I didn't reconnect with Source until I got a handle on my addictions at Alcoholics Anonymous through their surprisingly spiritual program.

When I started meditating, the door to Source opened more widely, and I began having visions and conversations with Jesus and the Madonna again, just as I'd had when I was a child. During this time, I was studying meditation with a Hindu seer and living in an ashram, but that didn't faze my powerful spiritual guides. Even when they were alive, Jesus and Mary knew that all traditions led to enlightenment. It doesn't matter what your beliefs are—Eastern, Western, or something in between that you've designed yourself—all that matters is that you are devoted and

93

consistent in your practices, because, ultimately, they all lead to the same place.

One day I was sitting in the early-morning darkness in one of the California mission churches, where I could feel the support of the spirits of deceased American Indians (who were far more connected and holy, by the way, than the priests who had presumed to teach them). It's pretty much a custom in such places not to disturb anyone who appears to be in prayer, so I was surprised to feel a tap on my shoulder. I opened my eyes and, to my astonishment, saw a very small, incredibly wrinkled nun dressed in traditional Carmelite garb. She appeared to be at least 70 years old and, I noticed, was missing most of her teeth.

She said, "I'm so sorry to disturb you, my dear, and I have no idea why I'm doing this, but I feel compelled to ask you if you'd like to go with me to see an apparition of the Virgin Mary."

What an opportunity! I followed her out of the church. Once we were outside, she explained that there was a woman living about an hour away who had visitations from the Madonna every day at 4 P.M. sharp, and this had been going on for more than five years. The Vatican had even sent an emissary to check it out and found it valid, which is quite significant because they are extremely conservative in their acknowledgment of Marian (related to Mary) sightings.

I met the sister back at the mission in the middle of the afternoon and followed her an hour north to a professional plaza where there were about 50 people in what appeared to be some kind of an office—hardly an auspicious location for an apparition. We arrived a few minutes late, and the people there were all fingering rosaries, which are prayer beads from ancient times. They were kneeling behind an unusually small woman at the front of the room who was also kneeling with her back to us. I was pretty skeptical; instead of getting down on my knees, too, I went to the back of the room and leaned against a filing cabinet.

As I looked out the window and wondered whether this whole thing was bogus, I suddenly felt a big shift of energy in the room, one of the biggest I'd ever felt—and at this point in my spiritual practice I was pretty experienced in the energy field. A bright light hit my eyes, I was thrown to my knees, and I was suddenly overwhelmed by the smell of roses. I never saw the Madonna, but I could definitely feel her. It was one of the strongest energy fields I'd ever experienced.

Without effort, I found myself in a state of exaltation, the result of those lengthy meditation sessions I'd been doing. If you read any of the spiritual masters, in any tradition from East to West, you'll find that euphoric sensation is a natural outgrowth of deep meditation.

The next thing I knew, the little woman at the front of the room appeared to be beckoning in my direction. "She means me?" I mouthed to those around me who had obviously been there before. They gestured that I was to go up and kneel next to her. Once I did, she and the Madonna, whose energy I could sense directly in front of me, had a conversation that I was not privy to while the woman gently touched different parts of my face and arms. I could tell that she was in an altered state.

After several minutes, the woman let me know that it was time for me to return back to my place. She beckoned a couple of other people and worked with them in a similar fashion. Another few minutes passed, and then I felt the energy shift back to normal while the light and scent of roses faded. The little gal went into a side room, and everything felt very flat and one-dimensional. The Madonna had definitely left the building.

I was overwhelmed by gratitude for the nun who had invited me, and I thanked her effusively. "Sister, I want you to know this was very valid!"

She retorted, "I already know that!" Obviously, she didn't need me to validate her experience!

After about ten minutes, the woman who had communicated with the Madonna came back into the room and read from something she had just written. She said, "The Madonna has asked me to write down what she said to me privately and come back in here and read it out loud. The person in the room for whose benefit it is will know it is for him or her." She kept her gaze down and never made eye contact with any of us . . . but the piece she read was obviously for me. I knew it, and so did the others in the room, but none of us spoke of it. It was a very private message, mostly a caution about the dangers of pride and the risks inherent in gaining any of the spiritual gifts, especially the gift of healing.

Afterward, I learned that each person in the room had had a different experience of the Madonna: some people could see her; some, like myself, could feel her; and some could hear her. All definitely sensed her presence.

I also learned that the little gal who was having these daily apparitions was small because she had been born with a birth defect that kept her from growing to full height. She was only about four and a half feet tall and had other related health problems. Although she looked a bit like a child, she was actually in her 40s. Formerly a nun living in a convent, she'd had to leave because she had so many health problems that the other nuns simply couldn't care for her anymore. As a result, this woman who was communicating with the Divine Feminine had taken a job washing windows and sweeping floors at McDonald's part-time. She is one of the best examples that supports my constant refrain: if you make lemonade out of the lemons that life gives you, you will indeed fulfill your purpose.

My consistent meditation and prayer practice had laid the groundwork for connecting so directly with the Madonna that day, and that encounter took me up another few levels energetically. Every time you tap into a force field that's considerably higher than your own, you automatically get pulled up, too. That's the reason why people who are striving to raise themselves spiritually like to go and sit at the feet of their master or, even better, touch them. That's the basis for the entire guru system in India.

The Only Life That Matters

Earlier in the book, I touched upon getting information from past lives, and I'd like to make one point about reincarnation and the importance of focusing on *this* lifetime as the only place to work through personal issues. What I've found when I contact those who have passed on is that they are often in a state of limbo. When I tune in to those who are deceased—which is as easy to do as it is to connect with someone who's alive—some of them seem to be stuck in between realities. Often, they think they are still alive and battling the same old "stuff" they worked on here. That is definitely something you want to steer clear of, unless you think being in your own version of the film *Groundhog Day* seems like a good idea.

The best way to avoid that is to figure out what your key life issues are. Then journal and meditate, meditate and journal, to stay as transparent as possible about your own stuff. Be sure to process it while you're here so that you don't have to spend eons in some twilight state figuring it out. And since time doesn't exist on the other planes, it *can* seem like an eternity! These tools are too simple not to use, and they will profoundly affect your experience of life now and your evolution as a soul.

Practice #3: Prayer

Prayer is another essential tool for connecting to Source and accessing its infinite capacity to heal. While it may never find its way into the *Physicians' Desk Reference*, distance healing and remote intercessory prayer have been verified by some scientific studies. For many of us, the idea of using prayer as a healing practice is distorted by the image of employing it to plead with an external deity. But when the practice is removed from any religious trappings and performed correctly, it becomes a profound way to generate healing. When a clear and loving intention is formed in the mind, held in the heart, and directed as prayer, it can have an amazing, therapeutic effect.

Whatever the concerns of your life, bring them into the cave of your heart (called the *hridayam* in Sanskrit) and the light of your higher self. Visualize doing this with intentional focus for a period of a few weeks, and the presence of Source will flow through you as easily as electricity flows through a lamp in your house. Flip the switch, turn on your heart and mind to love and gratitude, and the current will move through you.

When you are centered in your heart, you can begin to effect healing on the physical level. Start small: help resolve a disagreement, or calm your child down when she's afraid. See how your focused intent on bringing love to a situation through the heart can create a positive energy shift.

It's important to know that your mind and thoughts have a say in the future. You are a creator of this world. You came here to contribute to the betterment of all. There are a vast number of ways that you can serve to lift humanity out of the lower frequencies that feed fear, greed, and violence. It is in your hands to generate a better world through the power of the heart in alignment with a focused mind. This is prayer.

When you align with the love in your heart through prayer, you will immediately begin to see life differently. It creates movement not only in your thoughts, but also in your entire energy field. Align with your essential self, align with the infinite possibilities, and move from your heart center outward. The ripple effect will continue expanding in all directions.

These days, the kind of change that may have taken 20 years or even a lifetime in the past happens at a far more accelerated pace because time is speeding up. You've felt it, haven't you? This quickening allows rapid personal transformation. The physical world can shape-shift before your eyes when you are in deep alignment with All That Is, and the love and gratitude invoked through prayer can move mountains.

Practice #4: Forgiveness

One of the mountains that journaling, meditation, and prayer will help move is any energetic block we have inside that comes from holding on to anger and resentment. Forgiveness is perhaps the most important part of healing. When we suffer a wrong, or even a perceived wrong, we can harbor hatred and bitterness. This can be caused by abuse, abandonment, betrayal, divorce, death, and other hurtful situations that we never resolve. Not only can this discord cause illness (the heart chakra is associated with ailments ranging from asthma and pneumonia to lung and breast cancer), it can impede our progress toward healing.

Holding on to resentments and anger can ruin your quality of life. The only person who suffers from your failure to forgive is *you*—it is not the other guy. When you stay hostile or resentful, it tears down your immune system and increases your risk of disease. Get some help if you are troubled by a situation like a bad divorce or a child who went sideways. Whatever the circumstance is in your life, you can let go of it. Also, forgive yourself for whatever unhealthy lifestyle or emotional baggage you feel may have precipitated a disease. Self-blame doesn't help in healing.

Worrying about disease, let alone having one, often makes us want to find someone or something to blame. We blame our genes, our lifestyle, our job, our partner, ourselves.

It is so important to know that any disease you get, especially cancer, *is not your fault*. You did the best you could with what you knew then. There is no way to go back and undo any of the factors, such as inherited genes or exposure to pollutants or synthetic hormones. Guilt only compounds the problem, causing more emotional stress and disrupting the healing process. Therefore, one of the most powerful techniques you can use is the simple practice of forgiveness.

It is only today that you can change anything. Take a deep breath and decide that you are going to let go of any connection to an external cause. The only advantage to knowing about pollutants is if it helps you minimize your risk today, like stopping smoking or eating right. Instead of feeling despair and anguish, be hopeful for your own healing progress. Your body may be telling you that something is out of balance, that something more fundamental is wrong, but it is also telling you that you have the key to getting better.

When my husband, Eric, and I were rock climbing one day, he had a terrible fall off of a mountain and sustained what's called a "closed head injury," which means it is essentially untreatable. He went back into the hospital several times before we finally understood that nothing could be done. At the end of the first year, his condition had worsened. He couldn't walk or ride in a car, sit comfortably to read or watch television, or, on most days, even be civil. Sleep eluded him. Almost anything could set off a pattern of symptoms ranging from fits of choking—when I was certain he would die in my arms—to fits of rage and deep descents into depression. Any kind of mental or physical stimulation was completely out of the question. To add to the stress, we had no savings, no health insurance, and stacks and stacks of medical bills.

With Eric's condition so fragile, no one thought to ask how *I* was doing. As is so common with adults who were abused as children, I blamed myself for Eric's accident even though I was really not at fault. He and I had simply ignored the climber's maxim: "There are old climbers and there are bold climbers, but there are no old, bold climbers." We had climbed recklessly, and our luck had finally run out. Nevertheless, I was convinced that somehow I was responsible for this nearly fatal accident.

Within a matter of weeks after his fall, I developed an embarrassing speech impediment. I would open my mouth to speak and hear the words in my head, but nothing would come out except for a little croak. I also found it difficult to drive, as I was sure an accident was waiting around every corner. My food allergies intensified overnight, and I lost more than 30 pounds. By the end of that first year, I had some ominous symptoms that even I could not ignore, so I scheduled an appointment with a doctor. I was so distraught by the time I walked into her office that when she patted me gently on the arm, I began rocking back and forth in the chair, crying hysterically, and telling her, "I don't have a head injury! I don't have a head injury!"

At times when I was certain that Eric was resting comfortably, I went out for a walk in the nearby woods. Instinctively realizing that I needed to forgive myself because I was making myself sick, I felt compelled to pray in a low tone, saying over and over as if repeating a mantra, "You have been forgiven. You have been forgiven." I never questioned what this might mean, nor did I seek any other help. As it turned out, the more I prayed, the better I felt.

About the same time, I serendipitously stumbled upon a book by Louise Hay called *You Can Heal Your Life*. In fact, this book *saved* my life. From it, I formed the practice of saying positive affirmations (really, another way to pray), which helped me more fully forgive myself.

Ultimately, after many years of my performing healing treatments on my husband, as well as taking him for treatments administered by others in the field of alternative medicine, he finally made a complete recovery. Looking back on it now, I am truly grateful for the lesson the accident taught me about the incredible power of forgiveness.

Nearly every religion teaches that forgiveness is a virtue. As Alexander Pope said: "To err is human, to forgive divine." What ancient cultures have known for millennia is now becoming accepted by Western medicine. Numerous studies have found links between forgiveness and health, showing that pain levels decrease when patients used meditation techniques to forgive and release inner hurt. Research has also suggested that forgiving others and yourself can improve the functioning of your immune system.

Finally, let's be clear about what forgiveness is and what it is not. Forgiving others does *not* mean that you excuse what someone did to you. It means that you let go of the bitterness and negativity you are holding inside. It means that you let go of your need for revenge or retribution.

Many people equate forgiveness with weakness, thinking that it involves forgetting what has happened. For true healing, however, forgetting is as detrimental as not forgiving. You need to process what has happened, experience your emotions, and then find the strength to move on from there. Forgetting—burying the pain—will only cause disruption in your mind, body, and spirit. The important thing to remember is that it is for *you* that you forgive.

Sometimes individuals who have been diagnosed as terminal may feel: *I have so little time left, and I don't want to be angry and depressed and bitter anymore.* So they let go of those old feelings, and they start to talk to people whom they might have shut out of their lives for many years. Sometimes they even go on to have a remission.

EXERCISE: Hawaiian *ho pi'no pi'no*

This potent Hawaiian clearing technique activates forgiveness.

1. Choose any relationship that's ever troubled you. It could be one you're currently having with a family member—a parent, sibling, or child—or with someone who's deceased. It doesn't matter if the person is alive or if they've passed, because energetically we're all still connected.

2. Sitting comfortably with your eyes closed, bring that person into your mind's eye and place his or her image in front of you—3 or 4 feet away if your feelings about this individual were reasonably good, and 10 or 15 feet away if it was a very strained relationship. Now you're going to speak to this person, which will clarify, refine, and clear that relationship.

3. Start by doing the Microcosmic Orbit exercise that's found earlier in this chapter. During the energy's orbit, as you visualize it moving up your back and up to the pineal, breathe in and say in your mind to the person you have

chosen, "I'm sorry, forgive me." Then, as you exhale and move energy down the front of your body, say in your mind to that person, "I love you, thank you." It doesn't matter if you were 100 percent right or 100 percent wrong in all of the problems you had in this relationship. It doesn't make a bit of difference because here you're giving this person back his or her energy and receiving yours in return the same moment you are clearing it.

Remember to breathe in on the way up and out on the way down. Breathing in, as energy is going up the back, say, "I'm sorry, forgive me." Breathing out on its way down the front, it's "I love you, thank you." "I'm sorry, forgive me; I love you, thank you." "I'm sorry, forgive me; I love you, thank you."

If you find yourself getting very emotional while doing this forgiveness exercise, that's wonderful. It means that you are clearing those old emotions and healing the pain of that relationship.

The Legacy of Forgiveness

Forgiving can be tremendously difficult; and for victims of incest, severe abuse, and violence, it may seem impossible. Probably the hardest thing to forgive is the murder of your child. In August 1993, 26-year-old Amy Biehl, a Stanford graduate and Fulbright scholar who had been working against apartheid for a year in South Africa, was only days away from returning to the U.S. when she was stabbed, beaten, and stoned to death by angry young men who knew only that she was white. These days, through the extraordinary forgiveness of Amy's parents, two of the men who murdered their daughter work for the charity they founded in South Africa after she was killed.

Linda Biehl and her late husband, Peter, started the Amy Biehl Foundation a year after Amy's death with donations that had been sent by strangers. They quit their jobs to work full-time on racial reconciliation, and testified in favor of amnesty for the killers at the Truth and Reconciliation Commission. Desmond Tutu told them to speak from their hearts, and they did so. "It's liberating to forgive. We can sleep at night, and we feel totally at peace," Peter said.

Today, the foundation runs a range of programs—in health and safety, education, and arts and music—all aimed at preventing violence in the townships and squatter camps that sprang up during apartheid. Linda Biehl, astonishingly, travels the world with one of Amy's killers, telling her daughter's story and teaching about the tremendous healing power of forgiveness.

Practice #5: Being of Service

You can do everything in your power to journal away your energy blocks, meditate for hours a day to expand your consciousness, pray fervently, and seek and give forgiveness; but if you aren't being of service, it's all for naught. The same is true in reverse: if you are spending all of your time tirelessly in service to others and not doing the inner practices, you are also out of balance. There has to be an inner and outer harmony in your life to be an effective shaman, whether you are interested in healing only yourself or if you want to be able to work with others.

Being of service is not as scary as it may sound. You don't have to drop everything in your life and run off to a faraway location to help the victims of the latest natural disaster. Using the woman who channeled the Madonna and cleaned windows at McDonald's as an example, you are of service by doing whatever it is that you do, as long as you do it with love. Being of service, and doing it with the right attitude, means that what you do in some way elevates the people around you. Windows that are clean, after all, let in more light. Even if you're in one of the "helping" professions, you are really only being of service if you do your job in a compassionate way, alleviating the fear and pain of those who come to you. If you are so full of ego, anger, or bitterness that you are sending out negative energy, how much are you actually helping others?

Look carefully at what you "do" in the outer world. You constantly have the opportunity to be of service to every single person you meet throughout the course of your day. Smile at the harried checkout clerk in the supermarket; don't be pushy or rude to the people standing in line with you at the bank; don't take out your frustration on your kids, partner, or employees; and be generous and let that other car into the lane ahead of you! You are being of service each time you send out a current of caring for others, which clears space for you to receive more of the expanded energy of higher consciousness that you seek.

Your feet will fly along the path of the shaman when both directions—what comes in and what goes out—are in balance in your life.

Journaling, meditation, prayer, forgiveness, and being of service are staples for anyone who desires to be his or her own shaman and effect healing transformations in others. They are the quintessential tools for readying yourself for more advanced healing techniques.

Before we begin to look at what some of those methods might be, let's take a trip into the dark side of humanity so you'll know how to deal with that when you encounter it.

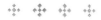

chapter seven

Psychic Warfare

Every single person on this planet, including you and me, has a dark side, which some call the "shadow." But where does it come from?

The dark side is a collection of your negative feelings—about yourself, your life, and others—that you haven't yet brought to consciousness and processed. The problem is that the majority of people aren't conscious of most of their thoughts, and this is why the path to becoming a healer needs to include meditation and journaling—two of the best tools for getting in contact with how you really feel and then attending to those emotions.

When we act from our shadow, we come from a place of negative energy, which in turn attracts the dark forces from beyond just like a magnet pulls iron filings to it. If we come from our own negativity often enough, we can become connected to that force. In extreme cases, we may even be possessed by it. As with everything else in life, we aren't helpless victims of our dark side—we always play a role in what happens to us. But we do have to be aware that others with whom we interact may be harboring such deep shadows that they have become evil.

Of course, we'd all like to pretend that wickedness doesn't exist. The evil eye, hexes, demonic possession—didn't they all go out with the Dark Ages? Unfortunately, evil is as real and prevalent today as at any other time in history.

You see, we all have the capacity for malevolence if we let our shadow side take over. When we become split from our own negative feelings, especially jealousy, our dark side can get in the driver's seat. At that point, we may not have any idea of the damage we are doing to others, but those who are intuitive will be able to sense it.

Have you run into problems caused by another person's negative intent? Maybe with a member of your own family? Stereotypes like the mother-in-law hell-bent on disempowering her son's wife are based on the reality of powerful, suppressed emotions such as jealousy.

Do you have a chronic health problem, such as headaches or backaches? Do you seem to come down with every virus in the neighborhood? Did your investments all go south with Bernie Madoff or any of the other money scoundrels? Some of your problems may be, in fact, caused by the negative intent of others—and I call that being under *psychic attack*.

Psychic attack happens when another person has formed an intention, consciously or not, to hurt you, and his or her negative energy has entered your own field and body. It can be as simple as picking up a little negative energy from someone who's in a bad mood, such as the bank teller or supermarket clerk who's having a bad day, or being stalked by a spurned lover—and can go all the way up to full-blown demonic possession.

People always ask me about possession, and I can tell you that I do not take it lightly. I know from experience how dangerous it is, and I'm always extremely careful when dealing with it. This is definitely one of the hardest things I work with as a healer.

How do you know if *you're* under psychic attack? Maybe you wake up with sciatica that won't go away, suddenly feel depressed for no reason at all, or feel totally stuck no matter what you do. Any of these examples can be evidence of a recent psychic attack. If you've had long-term problems that you haven't been able to track to their source, such as relationship issues or financial troubles or nagging health problems that have lasted for years, these may well be the result of psychic attacks from much earlier in life, possibly from childhood.

My own childhood experiences of the mother from hell, the incestuous father, and the pedophile priest laid the groundwork for my knowing how to recognize and deal with dark forces.

Doing Battle with Evil

I had spent many years working with shamans and healers and was fairly well versed in dealing with dark energies when I had a dark experience of my own one day. Seemingly for no reason at all, my back went out, and I was laid up in bed for a couple of weeks. I was in so much pain that I had to plead with various practitioners to make house calls to try to help me—from a chiropractor to an osteopath to an acupuncturist to an energy healer—but despite the numerous treatments, my situation didn't get any better.

After lying flat for more than two weeks, doing nothing except meditating and journaling and sleeping, I was getting really clear about the emotional issues I was working through as well as connecting with my guides. Then one night, I woke up and absolutely knew that there was a very dark energy in the right-hand corner of the ceiling in my room. I had never felt anything this profoundly evil and terrifying, and every hair on my body was standing straight up. It felt like something out of *Rosemary's Baby*. This accumulation of darkness actually spoke to me, saying, "If you'll give up your guides and join us, you'll get everything you want."

This was at a time in my life when all I wanted was to be able to heal others. I was deeply involved in this work in my private practice and in my teaching of healing techniques, but despite what seemed like a lifetime of effort, I hadn't ever accomplished much in the way of real physical healings. It was pretty discouraging, so you can imagine how tempting the darkness's offer was. All I had to do was join this energy and healings would start to happen.

I fought off the temptation, knowing that the trade-off was not one I was willing to make, and turned on the light next to my bed. On my nightstand was an icon of the main guide I work with. I held this image up toward the ceiling and demanded that, in His name, this energy leave immediately. The evil forces pulled backed a little but stayed in the room until dawn, making noise, rocking my bed, and scaring me half to death. They came back the next night, too.

During the day, I meditated and prayed on how to get rid of them. When they came back on the third night, I was ready. Despite the extreme back pain, I made myself stand up and face them. I had figured out that my injury was an illusion, although a very painful one! Armed with this realization, I had much more strength to stand and face this unwanted spirit. With the icon of my guide in one hand and a bottle of water I had blessed in His name in the other, I used fierce, unbending intent—a technique I had learned from a South American shaman—and ordered this evil power out of my room and out of my life. It worked!

Since then, the dark side has continued to test me periodically, but not as brazenly as that first time. Ultimately, I began to effect real healings, but ones that came from the Light, not the Dark. I remind myself each and every day that healing is a power, and power corrupts. If you're hoping to do this work, it's crucial that you start to understand this as well.

Now, I don't want you to start worrying that you're going to begin seeing evil forces on the ceiling of your bedroom—my experience was pretty unusual. But it was one more step on my path of learning how to help others release their dark energies. Today, I can clearly recognize the destructive qualities in others, and I know how to deal with them.

Have You Ever Been Slimed?

By far the most common and low-level kind of psychic attack happens when someone "slimes" you with his or her energy. The person sends out a negative thought or feeling, consciously or not, and if you have a hole in your energy field, it slips right in. This is a fairly ordinary energetic problem. Your field is a little like a house: the odd-numbered chakras and structured levels of your field (1, 3, 5, and 7) are like the walls; while the even-numbered chakras and unstructured levels of the field (2, 4, and 6) are more like the rooms. Consequently, negative energy will fill the rooms—the unstructured areas—first, since they are open space.

So this negative energy, or slime, fills your energy field and chakras and throws you off-kilter, perhaps making you feel emotional and triggering your unprocessed childhood issues. For example, if as a child you felt rejected and haven't yet resolved this issue, you may feel rejected now. That would be a second-chakra issue and may present itself as a food addiction.

If as a child you felt unloved and haven't come to terms with that, the slime may trigger these feelings in the present, which is a fourth-chakra issue that might surface as a chest cold. Or maybe you felt stupid as a child and haven't processed this yet. Well, chances are that this slime is making you feel stupid and dense and blank now. This is a sixth-chakra issue that might manifest as a headache.

All it takes is to have a short phone conversation with somebody who had an ax to grind, run into a friend who was jealous or resentful, or receive negative energy without even an e-mail or phone call, and the next thing you know you feel terrible and can't function right and have no idea why. These are examples of a low-level psychic attack.

Here's the solution: If you think you've been slimed, chances are you have. You can remove the negative energy that's in your body and energy field by adding one pound of sea salt and one pound of baking soda to a bath and soaking for 20 minutes. (I'll go into more detail about this later in the chapter.) Other possible solutions are to go for a swim in the ocean or spend 20 minutes sunbathing, preferably full body. If you feel fine afterward, it was slime; if you don't, it's more likely a cord.

The Cords That Connect Us

One of the most frequent methods of committing psychic warfare on another person is through energetic cording. *Cords* are streamers of auric light that connect us to one another, and each one matches up to the same chakra in the other person. (In other words, my third chakra would send a cord to your third chakra.) As you might suspect, there are good cords and there are bad cords. Good cords, for example, are the kind you got from your parents when they sent respect and care from their third chakra to your third chakra, or love from their heart chakra to yours.

The existence of negative cords indicates a vulnerability within us. If we can be negatively corded, it means that we have emotions we haven't processed, memories we haven't brought to closure. Again, that's why I'm always stressing the importance of meditation, journaling, therapy, and personal work. We cannot leave our "stuff"—our feelings about difficult experiences from the past—unresolved, because it leaves us susceptible to this type of psychic attack and wreaks havoc on our lives.

I once worked with a gal named Peggy who's a great example of this. She had finished writing portions of her first book, a memoir, and realized that the draft needed editing. She hired her friend Maria, who was an editor. What Peggy didn't know was that Maria had always dreamed of writing and publishing a book of her own. The more Maria worked on Peggy's draft, the more jealous she became of the natural writing talent she recognized in her friend's work. Bottom line: Maria wanted what Peggy had.

Maria's shadow side (remember, we all have one) wanted her friend to fail. Of course, Peggy wasn't aware of any of this. All she knew was that after about two weeks of having Maria work on her book, and despite the fact that they were living thousands of miles apart and only communicated via e-mail, she woke up one morning with writer's block and seemed to have lost all faith in her own ability to finish the manuscript. When this state didn't pass after several months, Peggy came to one of my workshops for help. The cause of her block was obvious: a cord from Maria's fifth chakra was sending negative energy into Peggy's fifth chakra, effectively shutting down her creativity and blocking her writing talent.

Anytime we're feeling a lack of confidence or enthusiasm for something positive we'd like to pursue, or find ourselves somehow sabotaging our own success, we must ask ourselves if we've made an unspoken cording agreement with someone else to not fully shine. We often make these agreements with our families because we don't want our parents or siblings or partners or children to feel bad about themselves in comparison to us, which then only results in keeping us small.

I removed the negative cord from Peggy, which sent the energy back to Maria, where it remains her issue to resolve. I also taught Peggy a shamanic technique right then and there that would help her regain her power (you'll be learning it later in this chapter, too). Practicing this method, she immediately felt lighter and freer. She got in touch with me later and said that she had hired a different editor and was writing again.

Cords can only be formed with the consent of both people involved; to that end, our consciousness accepts our parents' cords even prenatally. Looking back at Peggy and Maria, they had formed cords as friends through the heart chakra. Then, when Maria became jealous, she added a negative one to hurt her friend.

One cording experience you may have had is during the breakup of a romantic relationship. Did it feel as if something were being ripped out of your heart? That's the feeling when someone pulls back a good cord that was connected to one of your chakras. That painful memory of a lover leaving you, and a good cord being detached as a result, is evidence of just how significant these situations can be.

My experience with negative cords has been quite intense. My father, whom I adored, had corded me positively with love in my heart chakra. However, when he sexually abused me, this created a dark cord from his second chakra to mine, which robbed me of my innocence as a child. The molestation also formed a negative cord from his third chakra to mine, taking away my power and substituting his own—a result that comes with any kind of abuse.

While I was always consciously aware of my father's love for me, evinced by the positive heart-chakra cord, I was totally unaware of his bad cords until I became proficient as a healer and learned to disconnect them. Fortunately, when you cut a negative cord, it does not disturb any positive ones that originate from that person.

As you might expect, I also had negative cording from my mother as a child. She was jealous of my relationship with my father, and she corded the heck out of my third chakra in an effort to disempower me. She also corded me in my fifth chakra to keep me silent. It was rough!

The silver lining is that having to undo that negative cording made me very strong and extremely attuned to dark energy. I can not only sense these forces in other people and trace them back to their ugly source, but I can also often successfully return them to their sender.

Normally, there are supposed to be relational cords between the chakras of parents and their children. Then, as the young ones mature, the cords do, too. The health of any relationships you have can be determined by looking at, and feeling into, your cords. But the negative ones I described, between my parents and me and between Maria and Peggy, needed to be removed.

One of the most disturbing experiences I ever had as an adult was the result of my not having yet uncorded myself from my mother. Although I had completely worked my way through the many traumas with my father and had forgiven him, I simply didn't want to face the truth about my mom's hatred of me. We all want to think that our mothers love us, so I continued to kid myself about that well into adulthood.

One day I became an apprentice to a powerful female shaman whom, frankly, I was wary of. I knew that she had allowed her power to corrupt her (her reputation for this was legendary), but I was thrilled by the love and attention she showered upon me. This woman became the mother I'd never had, which was where I was vulnerable; I convinced myself that I'd stay just for the "learning experience" and not allow myself to be corded. What a joke that turned out to be! Within only a few months, I was totally disempowered.

One day I had a major initiation (you'll learn what this is shortly) in her presence, and suddenly, in front of all of her students, I began accomplishing healings that were beyond her abilities. She was furious. Overnight, she went fully into her shadow side and was determined to stop me from ever working again. She came after me with the full force of her power, and what a fearful sight that was! At the last minute, though, she wavered, and instead sent some of her students to try to ruin me. Fortunately, I was able to defeat them and, again, came out of it stronger for having had the experience.

The lesson I learned, and I reiterate this to you here, is to never, *ever*, give your power away—not to anyone and not under any circumstance—as it sets you up for psychic attack. I give my students all of the tools and skills they need to be fully self-empowered to properly defend themselves against these warfare tactics.

With training, it is possible to learn to send back negative cords. You can also have them removed by someone like me. Either way, you will want to learn the following powerful shamanic technique that will bring back the energy you've spent in any relationship.

Recapitulation—a Shamanic Technique

The Peruvian-born author and anthropologist Carlos Castaneda wrote a series of books about his studies into Mesoamerican shamanism. There's a debate going on these days about whether Castaneda's stories of being directly trained by the Yaqui shaman don Juan Matus are factually accurate or embellished fiction, but for our purposes it really doesn't matter. I've learned through experience that the methods he lays out in his books do actually work.

The most important one for you to become familiar with is a process of clearing out past memories that Castaneda refers to as *recapitulation*. Or, as one of his students said, it is "the act of calling back the energy we have already spent in past actions." It not only retrieves the energy you have given away in your lifetime, it also clears you of the energetic deposits of others.

Using this amazing technique, you can reconnect to your own vital energy that is trapped in another place and time and bring it back to you. In short, you return to the moments of your life when you spent the energy, relive them in as much detail as possible as if you were actually there now, and then your energy will be released and restored to you. This allows you to turn the clock back, as what ages you the most is your loss of energy. This can be of tremendous importance to someone with a physical illness.

The recapitulation process eliminates and dissolves emotional connections—the basis of a psychic attack—so that you can become clear. I'm in total agreement with Castaneda on this point: it isn't the events themselves that interfere with our clarity; it's the emotions that are attached to them.

He tells the story of when he was initially taught recapitulation by don Juan. He was first told to make a list of absolutely every person he had ever known. What a difficult assignment! At his next meeting with the shaman, Castaneda was instructed to go sit in silence and recapitulate everyone on the list. It took him about a year. When he was finished, he returned to don Juan, thinking he would be praised. Instead, as the story goes, the shaman told him he had done the process incorrectly and sent him back to do it all over again!

It is a good idea to make a list of everyone you've met who you feel has had an impact on you, either positive or negative, and work your way through that list by recapitulating one or two people a day. Be sure to include your current partner, your family members, and anyone with whom you've ever had a sexual relationship, as they are likely among the subjects you most need to recapitulate. You will be surprised at the amount of energy and clarity you regain by completing this process, even if you only do it partially.

This version of recapitulation is called "the Sweeping Breath," as it is the breath that powers the process. Basically, while you're recalling a person in your mind, you breathe in and move your head from right to left, picking up any energy you spent in the relationship. As you breathe out, your head moves from left to right and ejects the remaining fragments of this individual's energy from your field.

EXERCISE: The Sweeping Breath

1. Invocation:

    - Sit in a chair with your knees apart to maintain a good connection with the ground through your first chakra. Preferably make contact with the floor barefoot, as there are important chakras on the soles of your feet. (If you are tired, either take a nap first or plan to do this process when you are more alert.)

    - Invoke, out loud or silently, your higher self and any spiritual masters, guides, angels, or other beings whom you resonate with and would like to have help you. Their assistance will make your process more powerful. I have found that invoking don Juan works especially well in the recapitulation process, but feel free to call upon any master who appeals to you.

2. Choose a person to recapitulate:

    - Select anyone in your life with whom you've interacted—your mother, father, partner, child, boss, friend, or ex-friend—alive or dead. It can be someone you love deeply or someone you can barely stand. Do not pick a person with whom you've had any interactions in which you were frightened for your safety, as that requires another more advanced form of this practice that I teach in my 21st Century Energy Medicine Program. (For more information on this program, see the Appendix.) But feel free to choose someone with whom you've had plenty of upsetting experiences.

- Close your eyes and mentally place the person you have chosen to recapitulate directly in front of you. Picture everything about him or her—face, hairstyle, body, and clothing. Take a few minutes to let this individual come into your awareness as clearly as possible.

- Next, intend to visualize this person's surroundings, the place and room he or she is in, and bring that into focus as much as possible. If this is difficult for you, don't worry, as it may still occur later when you're doing the breathwork portion of the exercise.

3. Begin the Sweeping Breath:

- Breathe in through your mouth as you turn your head from the center to the left, and exhale out of your mouth as you turn your head past the center and over to the right. After the first breath or two, switch to breathing through your nose. Maintain the image of the person you chose to recapitulate. You may notice that he or she comes into sharper focus, or you may recall certain events that you have forgotten. Keep your internal focus on this individual until it appears that there is nothing, emotionally or situationally, left to process. About 10 to 15 minutes per person is the right length of time. When you are new at this, it's not unusual to have to repeat the technique for the key people in your life in order to totally complete the energy exchange.

- The function of the breath in this practice is to restore energy. Shamans in this tradition teach that the human energy field contains cobweblike filaments that are projected out of the *luminous mass* (their name for the human energy field) and propelled by emotions. Therefore, every situation or interaction where feelings are involved is potentially draining to your energy field. By your breathing in from right to left while remembering a feeling, the breath picks up the filaments of your energy that were left at the scene. The exhalation breath from left to right ejects any filaments of the person you are remembering that still remain.

- By focusing on one individual at a time, you get a thorough retrieval of filaments and releasing of attached stagnant emotions that have weighed you down and depleted you. It is the life-giving nature of breath that endows this practice with its cleansing capacity.

4. Disconnect:

- In order to disconnect from the other person, do three sweeping motions with the head in the same pattern but with no breath. Then let your head come to rest in the center. This intentionally detaches you from the person you have been recapitulating. As the last step, this is crucial to the process, so be sure to always include it!

Advanced Recapitulation for Highly Charged Situations and Psychic Attack

If you've ever been physically, emotionally, or sexually abused; threatened with physical violence; harassed or stalked; or have been under any other kind of serious psychic attack, whether at work or at home—or from an ex, a family member, a boss, or a total stranger—the more advanced form of recapitulation is the process for you. It doesn't matter if the situation happened decades ago or is still going on today. This in-depth practice is taught in detail in my 21st Century Energy Medicine Program online and in workshops, where I can work with you as you learn it. (See the Appendix for more information on this program.)

How to Protect Yourself

Dealing with the dark side of life doesn't have to be difficult or frightening—you just need to know what to look for and how to protect yourself. As discussed earlier, it's key that you keep yourself as clear as possible through daily meditation and frequent journaling so that you are less vulnerable to external forces. Here are some simple guidelines for protecting yourself in any encounter you have:

— Form an intention every day to be protected by your guides. Connect with those who advise you, and ask them to cover your back. Really, it's that simple. The best way to form an intention when you're new at it is to write it down and then say it out loud. With practice, you'll be able to quickly do this mentally.

— If you're in a situation where you suspect someone may be sending negative energy your way, don't face that person head-on, but instead stand or sit at a 90-degree angle so that you are at his or her side. This protects you from a direct hit of energy, whether intentional or not. Since it's unconscious thoughts that usually do the most damage, positioning yourself in this manner can often keep you out of harm's way.

— Every time you have an unpleasant encounter, spend a few quiet minutes alone. Go inside yourself and ask whether you feel as if you got slimed. Ninety percent of the time, you'll immediately know if you did or not. If you suspect that you picked up some negative energy, take a clearing bath when you get home that night. Again, that recipe is one pound each of sea salt and baking soda. You'll want to mix the ingredients in a bath that is not too hot, but comfortable, and rest there for a minimum of 20 minutes. When you're done with your soak, drain the bathwater and shower yourself off, washing your hair, too. This will remove any energy you may have picked up from someone else. It will also make you feel very clear and rested, and you'll sleep well. Whether you've been exposed to negative energy or not, this bath is the ticket for whenever you're overworked—it cleanses and charges your field, and you'll feel totally refreshed the next day.

— In addition to a clearing bath, you can purify yourself and your room, even an entire house, by burning Epsom salts. This is an amazing tool, but you have to be very careful in its execution, as you don't want to burn yourself or start a fire.

Get a small ceramic or glass container with a handle—like an individual soup or serving bowl—and put in about one cup of Epsom salts. Then pour over it one-half to one teaspoonful of 150-proof alcohol, the kind that is too strong to drink, and light it with a long-handled lighter. Be sure to use an oven mitt to hold it, as the bowl will get very hot. Shake the container lightly as the burning Epsom salts purify the air. Also move it up and down in front of and behind your body, about four to six inches away for safety (it's best to have a helper do this step), and around the room.

When you cleanse the room, go from the floor to head height in every corner, being sure to include the glass windows, the paintings, and the furniture. Remember, proceed with caution, as the container will become very hot. When you're done, keep your eye on the salts until they're cool enough to touch with your finger before you dispose of them. For this clearing exercise to work, it's crucial that you follow these instructions precisely.

With intention, bathing, and clearing, you can protect yourself from the negative energy of others. If you think about it, you can probably already sense when you're around harmful forces; you can feel them in people as well as in rooms you enter. With the tips I've given you, you'll find that they're not that difficult to clear. With that, you are now ready to begin learning some techniques for working with others.

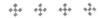

chapter eight

HEALING
TECHNIQUES

With the infinite universe as our toolbox, the resources available to us as aspiring healers are limitless.

Every culture throughout time has had its own unique system of healing. As I delved into the mysterious world of healers, sages, and shamans, I found myself being trained in a wide breadth of techniques. I was exposed to esoteric Christian modalities as well as Egyptian, Hindu, and shamanic schools of thought; all of this ultimately culminated in the development of a method of my own. Each approach I have learned has been based on principles of energy medicine and involved accessing Source—the unified field—and using every facet of our being to attract, conduct, and direct that energy to ourselves or others for the purpose of effecting transformation.

Since the sheer number of these techniques could fill volumes, my goal in this chapter is to give you a taste, a sampling, of the vast array that is available to the shaman. Some of them are accessible to you now in your current state of apprenticeship and can be learned from reading this book. Most methods, however, are far more complex and can only be mastered with many years of personal training under the guidance of a qualified instructor. Still,

I hope to spark your imagination as to what is possible for you as you begin walking the path of the shaman.

Let's start by learning about the Template of Perfection, which will allow for an intellectual understanding of what we seek to do as healers.

The Template of Perfection

Before our birth, we exist on a spiritual plane. When we decide to incarnate, that intention forms a template that encompasses our entire body and spirit and is perfect in every respect. The easiest way to picture this is as a blueprint of body and spirit.

As our life on Earth begins, and we're exposed to one trauma after another—from frightening experiences to abandonment to heartbreak—we drift away from being an exact replica of our Template of Perfection. Consequently, by the time we're adults, we may not resemble our original form at all. Whatever part of us is not peaceful and joyful won't match up to the Template. When we get far enough away from it, we often develop physical problems and disease.

When I was studying with the esoteric Christian group, I was learning how to bring people back to their Template of Perfection through prayer in order for them to heal. One day my teacher told me that I was ready to leave the academic setting, where everything was pure theory, and put my skills into practice—so she'd secured an invitation for me to work at their institution as a faith healer. My first day there, I found out that it's one thing to *think about* impressing a Template of Perfection on someone to such an extent that his or her body is healed . . . and quite another to actually accomplish it!

I was initially sent to a room at the facility and told simply to "pray about the condition of the occupant," and opened the door to find a very pretty woman who looked to be in her early 30s. After learning that she had no sensation below the waist, I assumed that she'd had some sort of spinal damage. However, in the tradition I was studying, it was very important that we never gave a problem a name so that neither we nor the patients bought into a medical diagnosis. (Consider how many times we catch ourselves identifying strongly with our own health problems, saying "my diabetes" or "my high blood pressure." This only signals to our body and mind that we are stuck with that issue.)

So here was this woman who couldn't move her legs. After a few minutes, I got over my initial fear and proceeded to spend days and days sitting at her bedside as I practiced focusing on a picture of her perfection in my mind's eye—walking, running, jumping, and so forth. I'm oversimplifying, of course, as I had spent more than several years before that learning how to form the kind of directed intention that could effect change at the cellular level. To make a long story short, this gal did begin to have some small but discernible movement before I was rotated to another room. I continued to work on my ability to impress a Template of Perfection on people for many, many years before having any real success.

These days, I intentionally create a Template of Perfection that covers everyone I'm with—whether in person, online, in teleconferences, during my radio show, or on TV. It doesn't matter what side of the world you're on, or whether you're listening or watching live or not, as my work is not circumscribed by time and space limitations—you are still covered by the Template of Perfection I've created. That Template automatically raises you to a higher vibratory level and brings you more in connection with the unified field, where every fact—past, present, and future—is available to you, as is perfect healing.

The most exciting thing for those wanting to become healers, the benefit of which I've been touting throughout this book, is that it's absolutely impossible to study this subject without being healed in the process. Every part of you that has separated from your own Template of Perfection, whether it's your emotions or your body or your soul, will come back into alignment as you learn how to heal others. If you're as goal oriented as I am, this should be irresistible—two accomplishments at one time!

Healing with Sound

One of the very earliest healing techniques in the history of the human race is healing through the use of sound. Prior to the written word, there was the spoken word, or sound, and ancient scriptures talk about its profound effect on our bodies, minds, and souls. Two religious texts that I am familiar with—the Bible from the Judeo-Christian world and the ancient texts of the Vedas—both refer to the power of sound to bring about change and transformation.

Your body and energy field operate in much the same way as an orchestra. Each of your chakras has its own vibrational frequency; together with the vibrations of your organs and emotional states, they work to create a symphony in your field. When you are in harmony, where everything is aligned and functioning optimally, that's called a state of *sound health.*

I'm sure you've had many positive and negative experiences with sound, from the pleasant resonance of nature (raindrops falling on wet leaves, the silence of snow falling, or the mad whirring of a hummingbird's wings)—to the most jarring of man-made noises (a partner screaming at you, a jackhammer pounding away on a nearby street, or heavy-metal music blaring so loud that it injures the fine mechanisms in your inner ears). You more than likely know firsthand how sound can both heal and destroy.

I spent some time in prayer in Benedictine cloisters at one point, and there I was trained to chant and pray aloud. I discovered that chanting, when done correctly, can alter our state of consciousness and bring us closer to spirit. The upsurge in popularity in the West of *kirtan*—the practice of chanting in the Hindu convention—shows the new openness to learning from these ancient traditions.

When I studied sound healing in Mystery School, I learned how to change the size and shape of a chakra by using a certain pitch vocally. I also received instruction on how to use sound to heal broken bones, scars, wounds, tumors, and the like. There isn't any medical condition that fails to respond to the trained use of sound. Think of the effect of music (entire books have been written on this subject) and how it can both transport and heal us.

My most memorable experience with sound happened some months after I began the practice of four-hour meditations every morning at a local chapel. Besides my study with healing masters, it was through these intensive and lengthy meditations that I developed my knowledge and skills for healing others and helping them along in their spiritual advancement. Developing the tool of *sounding* (releasing a spontaneous vocalization) was no different. Shortly after I began these extended periods of meditation and prayer, I found that I would begin sounding quite loudly on occasions when the person I was working with was about to move up spiritually to the next level. I intuitively knew that a certain tone would assist me in bringing in higher-level energy to transport him or her to that step up. It wasn't something I actually thought about, but rather something my body instinctively knew to do.

If you've got any reservations about making a fool of yourself in public, this practice will help you quickly get over that problem. There's nothing like sounding at the top of your lungs in front of thousands of people to cure you of any residual self-consciousness you might have! The first time I sounded in front of a large audience, I was fortunate enough to have a team of musicians on hand who promptly began to accompany me as I did so, which made me feel more comfortable. Today, I don't give it a second thought.

Sound healing is a complex topic, so I'd like to just bring your attention to its significance in your life. Which sounds please you the most? Which ones upset you the most? Which sounds can you simply not tolerate?

Try to set aside a little time each day to listen to the sounds you like, for those are the ones that heal you. So the next time you're relaxing at home, listening to the sounds of nature or music (as opposed to the leaf blower or lawn mower in your neighbor's yard), ask yourself what effect you think it is having on each of your chakras, from bottom to top. Jot down a few notes and then compare those responses to the next time you have a moment to consciously listen to pleasant sounds again.

I'm reminded of when I was on a book tour a couple of years ago, and I stayed in New York City for nearly a month. The hotel was reasonably quiet during the day, but every night at exactly 9 P.M. an enormous construction crew began work on the demolition of the hotel directly across the street. All I could hear were wrecking balls, along with huge cranes that continually made that high-pitched beeping sound when they backed up . . . and they didn't stop until exactly 5 A.M.

The noise completely disrupted my rest. After all, I'd come to the big city from the mountaintop I lived on, where I was used to hearing nothing but owls and coyotes crying in the night. I tried to hang in there and not complain, thinking it would be a good exercise in accepting what is, but after ten days I finally asked to be moved to the other side of the building. And I couldn't believe how much better I felt after only one night of decent rest. Don't discount the importance of serenity in your life; in fact, take a moment now to evaluate how much quiet you're getting. Is it enough?

At one point I studied music at a conservatory in Boston and they brought in a sound teacher from France. I got to spend an incredible weekend with this talented man. Without speaking, he made sounds and gestured for us to join in until we were having a conversation that seemed to make sense without words. By the end of the program, we were all spontaneously communicating in sound.

As I walked out of the workshop late on the last evening, a jet passed overhead, and I was able to hear a full orchestral chord in the sky from the noise it made! I had been so opened to sound by this amazing experience, and this is possible for you, too. All you have to do to become more aware of sound is to start consciously listening.

EXERCISE: Toning

How often have you thought, *I don't like the tone of her voice?* Or do you remember your parents ever uttering that famous command: "Watch your tone when you speak to me"? Every person's voice, every noise you hear, and every musical instrument has its own vibratory makeup that's as unique as your individual energy field. The tonal quality of a sound is based upon either the presence or lack of *harmonics,* which are the frequencies that give a sound its characteristics.

When you want to "tone down" the chaos of your day or mellow out your thoughts and emotions so you can meditate, get ready for your workday, or practice energy healing, you can give yourself a session of what is called *toning* by completing this exercise one or two times through. This will take you only a few minutes.

The seed syllable *om* is said to be the very first vibration that became sound—the *word* that was in the very beginning. It represents the union of body, mind, and spirit; so by intoning *om,* you are bringing yourself into harmony with All That Is.

Let's give it a try:

1. Stand comfortably, preferably in a quiet area, and take a minute to center yourself. Close your eyes so that you can concentrate on the sound of your voice.

2. Take a deep breath from your diaphragm, and imagine your body being filled with light as you breathe in. When you exhale, chant the sound of *om* for as long as your breath comfortably allows. Focus on the sound. Do this three times:

    Om . . . om . . . om

3. Take a moment to listen to your own sound, then chant *om* three more times.

Om . . . om . . . om

4. Open your eyes.

This process helps bring your body into resonance with itself—and you'll likely find that you experience more peace, energy, and vitality after just one session of toning.

Healing with Color

Similar to sound, color undoubtedly has an impact on your feelings and energy field; its vibrations affect you, and you can actually use it to heal yourself and others. Think about what colors you like to wear. When you have on your favorite hues, I bet you feel better and have a better day. That's because they're helping you self-heal.

As you deepen your practices of journaling, meditation, and prayer, you may start to see colors when you look at other people. Remember, it's not necessary to be clairvoyant to be a good healer, but keeping your mind open to being able to perceive colors gives you another source of information that can be used in healing. For instance, you may be able to discern that someone is projecting a dark red color, and what you're sensing is that deep down they are extremely angry, even if this doesn't show on the surface. It could be buried anger, for instance, and that could be helpful to know.

Conversely, you may be picking up the quality of red by "direct knowing," a by-product of a well functioning seventh chakra, as opposed to seeing it clairvoyantly. Picking things up through this type of direct knowing is more valid than clairvoyantly perceiving them because, as I mentioned, clairvoyant information can often be distorted or easily misinterpreted by the viewer. Most of the time, I personally rely on that which is received through direct knowing because of its trustworthiness. The best way to develop your direct-knowing capacity is to work with a teacher who can confirm or deny the accuracies of your perceptions; without that feedback, you may fall prey to "garbage in/garbage out" and simply be recycling your own, incorrect perceptions.

If the person seemed to be a lighter shade of red, like a rose color, and that made you feel all nice and warm inside, this means that his or her heart is open and loving. That's because it's a more positive shade than the darker red of anger. When you sense that someone is loving, you are likely receiving this information through your heart chakra. This feeling skill, as I mentioned earlier, is a very valid source, and the easiest channel to develop for most people. When combined with a direct knowing, you've got a double source of highly reliable information.

EXERCISE: Learning to Heal with Color

The following is a simple exercise you can do right now to begin healing with color:

1. Picture the rainbow and choose the color you like the best. See yourself dressed in that color. How does it make you feel? More or less powerful, happy, or peaceful?

2. Now think about another color and imagine yourself dressed in it. Do you feel different in this second hue?

3. Go back to your favorite color. Intend to project it from yourself to a friend or family member. How would that make him or her feel—powerful or weak, happy or depressed, peaceful or chaotic?

4. Once you learn to project colors, you can send them to others when you discern that their fields need particular ones in order to heal.

Adding Energy to Your System

One of the best places to start practicing healing techniques is on yourself. Try the following exercise the next time you're feeling lethargic or "off," since it will help you attract energy to your own field.

EXERCISE: Filling Your Chakras

- Close your eyes and bring your focus to your crown chakra, right at the very top of your head.

- Visualize it opening like the lotus flower it is so commonly associated with. As the flower opens, intend for a shower of energy to come down from the universe above and fill your crown chakra. Perhaps to you this will look like a shaft of light or feel like a warm breeze or a ray of sunshine. Know that you are being replenished with that energy from above.

- Now picture that energy overflowing your crown chakra and gently running down and filling your third eye (sixth chakra—between your eyebrows) then coming down to your throat. Pause for a moment there in your fifth chakra. Allow the energy to cascade down and fill your thymus, located just below the thyroid.

- Let it run down and accumulate in your heart chakra, located right in the center of your chest.

- Then allow it to bubble over and fill your solar plexus chakra, located above your waist.

- Next, let it run down and occupy your second chakra, halfway between your waist and your base chakra.

- Finally, let it flow into and fill your base chakra, located at the genitals.

- When you reach the base chakra, go back up to the top and repeat the sequence, allowing more and more of that inexhaustible supply of universal God-force to permeate your system. Picture it as a constant warm stream, simultaneously filling and clearing you. When you feel cleared and full, simply open your eyes, take a deep breath, and go back to your day.

When you've practiced this exercise a few times, you'll be ready to learn how to do the same sort of healing on others.

Psychic Surgery

One of the most controversial healing techniques in the world today, by far, is psychic surgery—it is a jaw-dropping experience to witness this phenomenon in action! In the healing field, the term *psychic surgery* has several meanings, depending on where you are in the world. In Brazil, where the practice developed in the 1950s and '60s as an outgrowth of a major spiritual movement, it is mixed with quite a bit of shamanic ritual originating from the African slaves and their descendants who have lived there since colonial times.

When I went to visit John of God, the most well known of the Brazilian psychic surgeons, I had almost no knowledge of his methods. I arrived just before he started one morning, and found myself in a very large open-air room with hundreds of people, all wearing white. Of course, everyone there spoke Portuguese, the language of Brazil, and there were several hours of speeches and prayer before John of God came into the room. I took the only seat I could find, and later was embarrassed to discover that I was sitting on the "stage." When he entered to begin his work, I was just a few feet from him.

The first thing I noticed was that John was in a self-induced trance and not conscious—which horrified me! I know how dangerous that is, as really bad things can happen when you completely vacate your body and allow other spirits to inhabit it. Nevertheless, I could sense that his consciousness was absent and the soul of a deceased physician was fully inhabiting his physical self and awareness.

A woman in her 40s was brought in from behind a curtain and stood up against a wall. John of God walked up to her, took a surgical tool from a tray that was held by a helper, faced the woman, pulled up her shirt and bra, and cut right into her breast. He then pulled what appeared to be a tumor out with his hands. The whole thing took a matter of seconds. I couldn't believe my eyes! The woman fell into the arms of assistants, who carried her backstage. I could both see and feel what John was doing, and it was definitely powerful, although there are no statistics available to validate the success of his treatments in curing either the physical or psychic ailments that people come to him for.

Without washing his hands or cleaning his knife, he proceeded to cut right into his next subject. Amazingly, despite the lack of sanitation, no infections have been reported in the recipients of John's psychic surgery.

While the psychic surgeons from Brazil and the Philippines are often quite connected to Source, their approaches are sometimes antiquated and often put them at risk. The healing techniques I teach are as revolutionary and exciting, but much safer for both healer and client.

Through *etheric template surgery*, the healer operates on the individual's energy field as opposed to his or her physical body the way a psychic surgeon does. This is an important basic technique to master prior to learning the advanced one that I developed, which involves working inside the physical body as opposed to the energy field.

To perform etheric template surgery, the healer must first know how to locate and enter the fifth level of the client's human energy field—the ability to stay on this level isn't a hard skill to learn. This fifth level is the template for the physical body; it looks just like the negative of a photograph. If part of your body goes haywire, balance needs to be reestablished in this area, the etheric template level, and then you can regain your healthy physical form.

Once you learn how to stay on the fifth level, which must be taught to you by a qualified teacher, you will be able to connect with the energy of deceased surgeons or other knowledgeable guides who do the surgery through you. If you're clairsentient, you'll be able to sense as the guides come into your energy field and send their instruments down your arms and into the client's field. It's an amazing experience as a healer, but can be extremely tiring. And please keep in mind that you have to stay completely conscious at all times in order to protect yourself and your own field from undesirable energies.

Walk In

One day, after many, many years of apprenticeship coupled with rigorous self-analysis, I was summoned by a shaman I had trained with some years before. He said that he had been given a message during his meditation that he was to assist in my transformation. I had no idea what he meant by that, but was intrigued and promptly made the journey to his remote area. As I entered his healing space, he gestured for me to lie on a mat. At first he said nothing, simply waving a large feather over me and humming in the tradition that he had taught me. I knew that he was checking my energy field. After a few minutes, he said, "I don't wish to frighten you, but you appear to be dying."

As you might expect, I didn't take this news lightly. I wasn't quite ready to leave; rather, I sensed that my life's work was just beginning. In fact, several months before he contacted me, I had begun to feel deeply that I was about to achieve a new level of healing.

A long period of silence ensued. Then the shaman said, "Ah, you have completed the goals of this incarnation. Your final goal was to conquer your pride, and you have accomplished that sooner than expected. You are free to leave now if you wish, but it feels as if you would prefer to reincarnate in the same body. Is that true?"

I replied that this was indeed the case! Frankly, I was in no mood to die. The shaman went on to explain to me that future lifetimes can, in certain limited circumstances, be taken on at the completion of this one if the future life is visible in the individual's energy field. He told me that he had only seen this phenomenon once before but could sense a matrix of energy around my spine that was the consciousness of the life I could elect to begin now, if I so chose.

I elected at that very moment to stay and reincarnate in this same body, and the shaman began the process of helping me integrate the burgeoning consciousness into my present consciousness so that I could allow it to "walk in," to use the popular vernacular. At first I felt odd, a bit like I was someone else, but after a while that sensation diminished. Within a year, I couldn't really discern any difference—it all felt like me.

At the same time, I noticed that my healing technique was now different. I had witnessed a drastic shift the day that I was working on Jennifer, the young woman with the brain tumor whom I talked about in Chapter 4. But this time the change was a lot more subtle—I sensed that I had "graduated" from the Mystery School arena. I mentally thanked all of those teachers and mentors and clients and students who had taught me and helped me practice all of those skills, but I realized that I would no longer need them.

I found myself going back to the pure practice of prayer that I had learned so well from the esoteric Christian healers coupled with the unbending intent I had attained with the South American shamans. Deeply connected to my guides, and through them to All That Is, I started to heal the way I do now: by connecting myself to a field of intentionality until I "become" that level of intentionality. Once there, I am able to use the limitless Source to reorganize energy at the level of your body, your personality, your soul. I teach this technique in my 21st Century Energy Medicine Program.

As you progress along your own path, you will find what does and does not work for you. Know that this may change as you become more adept in communicating with Source, learning from your own healing process and helping others.

You may also find that, as you dedicate yourself to traveling this path and deepen your connection to Source, you are able to receive and hold higher-level energies that step you up in consciousness. This is one of the most exciting aspects of becoming your own shaman, and it's the subject of the next chapter.

chapter nine

INITIATION

Life on Earth is about evolution. Our bodies evolve, of course, but much more important is the evolution of our *consciousness*. We are given this particular lifetime so that we may experience relationships—the greatest vessel for personal growth—to give us the opportunities needed to master the particular life lessons our souls have set out to learn.

Our consciousness is a part of that vast force field that is the Creator of All That Is. Some call it the unified field, Source, or Spirit, as I have done in this book; others use Oneness, The All, or God. You may have your own name for it.

Each of us is part of this omnipresent energy, even if we can't always see or feel it. We often have a yearning to connect to that Source, a homesickness that pulls us—perhaps that's why you're reading this book. Our ultimate goal, then, is to reach ever-higher levels of consciousness that bring us closer and closer to manifesting that God-force within. When an expansion of consciousness occurs rapidly, it's called an *initiation*.

Initiations have been a part of every religion and in every culture. Even though they're called different names, they all describe the same phenomenon. But even an initiatory experience of the One is only a momentary glimpse of a reality that, because it is infinite, is essentially unknowable in the human body.

Near-Death Experiences

One way to experience an initiation is through a near-death experience (NDE). For obvious reasons, this is certainly not the desired way; nevertheless, I've found it interesting to study NDEs for the information they offer about initiations.

We understand in our limited intellect a little about Oneness, but merging our consciousness with the absolute Source *cannot* be done mentally—it can only be realized by direct experience. And an NDE offers us just that.

It's been estimated that more than 13 million Americans have reported having had a near-death experience. The number of NDEs has jumped since we've been able to shock hearts back to life after they've stopped beating. But many different circumstances can create NDEs besides cardiac arrest, such as rapid blood loss, electrocution, near drownings, traumatic injuries to the brain, and suicide attempts.

What do people experience in an NDE? Most often, they feel detached from their body; and their fear is replaced by serenity, security, and warmth. Some sort of a life review may take place, and there is often a sensation of being in a tunnel that leads to the presence of a light or beings of light. Finally, individuals are told to return to life on Earth. This process is the same from culture to culture, except that the beings of light are those associated with the person's particular culture.

A First Date . . . and a Near-Death Experience

I've had more accidents than I can count, but I've only had one near-death experience. It happened when I was a student in law school and on a date with Eric, a mountain-climbing guide from France who spoke little English—and, as it turns out, he's the man I later married. Even though it was February, for our first date he wanted to take me on a "practice" climb. As I would soon find out, it was an inauspicious time of the year for this activity.

Being French, Eric drove like a madman up to winter snows high in the Sierra Nevada Mountains and parked next to the Cosumnes

River—an awesome sight as it frothed and foamed like a wild animal. He outfitted me in heavy climbing boots, a winter coat, and a 165-foot rope that he tied to my back. Then he started hiking very rapidly up the trail along the river, and I valiantly did my best to follow. Unfortunately, I didn't have any wilderness experience and I wasn't exactly physically fit back then (my obsession with mountain climbing and ski racing came later on). The one sport I had mastered was swimming, and as I hurried alongside this mighty river, I could see that it wasn't exactly swimmable.

As we got farther up the trail, the river completely disappeared under granite, sometimes for hundreds of feet, before it would reappear downstream. We then passed a good-sized waterfall. At one point, Eric must have decided to cross the river up ahead, as I could see him running across the granite. Attempting to keep him in sight, I too ran across the rock, but as I crossed the wet stones, I slipped and slid into a small pothole. For a moment, my shoulders caught and I thought I was safe, but a second later, I was pulled under.

I thought I was a goner as I was being tossed about like a rag doll in the underground river. I tried desperately to untie the climbing rope that was strapped to my back, fearing that it would catch on a submerged rock or tree limb, but it was hopeless in the freezing cold and strong current. I ran out of air and started to take in water, when suddenly my extreme panic shifted to an incredible state of calm. Despite the icy temperature, I started to feel warm and peaceful. With quite a bit of detachment, I saw the highlights of my short life pass before me. Then I heard a voice—which seemed to come from both within and without—saying, "Go back. You still have a lot to do." I suddenly surfaced in a pool above the big waterfall we had passed on the way in. I managed to scream, and a couple of nearby climbers threw me a rope and pulled me to shore. Meanwhile, Eric was upstream wondering what had happened to his date.

In the weeks and months that followed, I noticed that life looked somehow different. I felt a lot more love for myself and everyone I met, and I had a clearer sense of my true purpose. It wasn't until some years later that I realized I'd had an NDE.

Those of the scientific community, God bless 'em, are still trying to explain away NDEs, but I can assure you that they are real. Where scientists have been helpful is in reporting some common aftereffects of such experiences, which usually include shifts in personality, such as a greater appreciation for life, higher self-esteem, and more compassion for others. Other typical responses include a heightened sense of purpose, a desire to learn, elevated spirituality, and greater ecological sensitivity and planetary concern. Other changes reported are: being more intuitive; increased physical sensitivity; a diminished tolerance for light, alcohol, and drugs; and a feeling that a person's brain has been "altered" so that he or she is now using the whole brain rather than just a small part of it. Interestingly enough, many of these are the same developments that I've noticed in myself and in others following an initiation.

Likewise, what I've observed in working with tens of thousands of people, many of whom have experienced an initiation while with me, I've also noticed in the energy fields of those who have had an NDE: the chakras in both groups are much more open and vibrating at a higher energetic level. The good news is that NDEs are not the only way to step up spiritually—a regular meditation practice and doing everything you can to cheerfully deal with whatever life sends your way are far safer approaches to inviting a spiritual initiation.

Initiations Happen More Often These Days

When I was a Mystery School student, it was uncommon for someone to go through more than one initiation in a lifetime. And it wasn't unusual back then to see only a handful of students out of a class of 50 go through one during a four- or five-year program.

As I continued on my own journey in the healing world, and went from being a student to a teacher, it became apparent early on that I had a real knack for connecting to higher energy levels and helping others with their initiations. At first, I would only assist 2 or 3 individuals out of a group of 50. These days, I often initiate more than half of the people in a room of 1,000. On days when I'm really "on my game" and consciousness is already high in the participants, I can lift an entire room at once. Remember, every single person comes into this lifetime with a unique skill that can be brought out. This is one talent I happen to have, and you have a special talent that can be developed as well.

Since around the year 2000, I've noticed that more and more of us are ready to be initiated, and that some people can even go through several initiations in quick succession. I have a theory about why initiations are happening with so much more frequency: Spirit is aware that our world is in a real state of crisis, so we need as many conscious people as possible who are willing to be of service.

And, as we talked about in Chapter 6, don't think too narrowly about what *service* means. Whatever you are currently doing—and I don't care if it's cleaning toilets or pet sitting or fixing computers —you *can* be of service. In fact, it's often better for your spiritual development if your job is menial. If you're coming from your heart, carrying out your purpose with total love and surrender to the Divine Plan and the benefit of others, then you are doing your part to change the world.

I often have to give aspiring initiates the bad news that they are on the edge of the next level but lacking a sufficient base of meditation—one that can come from any tradition or source—for me to safely move them up. And I've found that meditation forms can vary. I vividly remember an initiation that a gal went through at a workshop, and her form of meditation was pole dancing! Remember, leave your limiting beliefs at the door. Spirit has no such restraints.

When I first started facilitating initiations, I found that they can be very physical for both the facilitator and the initiate. I also discovered that the more I helped people through the process, the better I got at it. The more I assisted, the easier it got for me to hold the space for those higher-level energies to enter, and the faster I was able to accomplish the initiations. This fits in well with my type A personality. By doing this work, I have found that Spirit has quite a sense of humor and makes use of our personalities with all of our eccentricities and peculiarities. After all, we are always human, no matter how many initiations we take.

The Levels of Initiation

An initiation means that our consciousness has been expanded to some degree. Before the first one, all we care about is ourselves. We're focused on survival and getting our desires fulfilled. We're pretty much wrapped up in our own bodies, and we are motivated by fear. I lived for a while on this level, only caring about how I looked and disempowering those around me. I call this my "size 2" period, where, as I've mentioned, I was obsessed with fitting into size-2 clothing.

You may have come into this lifetime with a few initiations already under your belt, with what's called an "old soul," and if you make the right choice each time Spirit offers you two roads, you will blast past the first few levels easily and be ready for higher ones.

Here's a quick glimpse at the levels of initiation:

— Once you go through the **first initiation,** you begin to have the desire to do good, realizing that there are other people around besides yourself. At this level, you develop an appreciation for nature, too. The eighth chakra (above the head), which is also called the *soul star,* begins to influence your pineal gland. What this means is that you now have the "juice," the connection to Source, to bring forth the higher qualities that your soul yearns for: courage, creativity, compassion, and so on.

The very fact that you are reading this book guarantees that you are already initiated to the first level or higher. You wouldn't have even the slightest interest in this material if you were closed off to Spirit and living your first lifetime, so to speak. Here's a simple test: if you have a desire to do good and you appreciate nature, you've already made it to the first level. So take a deep breath and know that you've already been initiated—you can stop worrying that you're not worthy.

— This may sound basic, but there is nothing without love—for the self and for others. The **second initiation** opens your heart to Divine love and begins your journey into self-responsibility. At this second level, individuals most often look outside of themselves for God, not yet realizing that this force is both within and without and that they are already deeply connected to it. In my experience, the thing that most often blocks people from taking the second initiation is dislike for themselves, which is extremely common and highly destructive.

The first- and second-level initiations can occur spontaneously and take place anywhere. They often happen without any fanfare and don't require a facilitator. Maybe you had one while making love, which can be one of the most spiritual experiences available to us humans; at the birth of a child; at the death of a loved one; or during a sudden *Aha!* moment—perhaps while walking in the woods, gardening, running, doing yoga, or sailing. It can be anything that gives you a moment where you see beyond your everyday me-me-me consciousness and realize the vastness to which you are connected.

— If you're doing your best with your life problems and don't resort to blaming others, being a victim, or going into bitterness or self-pity when things aren't the way you want them to be—and if you have a deep desire to help other people—there's a strong likelihood that you're ripe for a higher initiation, which usually requires a facilitator.

The **third initiation,** called the *soul merge,* is where the light of the soul star (the eighth chakra) fully downloads through the chakra system and anchors into the center of the earth. This is usually a pretty big deal and most often requires assistance. Finally, all of the energy, light, and consciousness of your soul merges with your physical body. This basically brings your soul to Earth and allows much more of you to be present in your body. You begin to experience what is called "soul-based consciousness," which means that every decision you make will henceforth be based on your higher qualities instead of your lower ones. (Again, for characteristics of the higher self, think courage versus timidity, unconditional love versus jealousy, generosity versus stinginess, and so forth.)

In this initiation, you start to become aware of your ego issues, and this is usually a very long process. It can take years of work to do everything that an expansion of consciousness makes available for you. An initiation simply puts you on the launchpad of the Divine—you have to do all of the hard work in order to actually take off.

— In the **fourth initiation,** the membrane of the soul star is absorbed into your 12th chakra, located far above your head. This can really be an ecstatic physical experience. Here's where your identification with your ego and personality really shifts to being soul based rather than personality based. The soul star releases its accumulated understandings from previous lifetimes, and your crown chakra opens more and is purified, preparing you for higher initiations where your consciousness can become reunited with God consciousness. At this point, you will be considered for acceptance into the Brotherhood of Light, the name used to encompass all of those who work for the Light as opposed to the Dark.

— In the **fifth initiation,** the light energy of the heart of the soul star is downloaded into your own heart, which activates the connection between your heart and thymus and your energy field and physical body. This is the first infusion of the Christ consciousness, or Christ light, and the beginning of solar consciousness. It blows open the heart chakra and purifies it, especially with regard to issues of worthiness.

I won't go into detail here on Levels 6 through 12 because they are fairly rare. If you'd like to know more, though, I cover them in detail in an article at **www.DeborahKingCenter.com/ resource/initiations.** These higher-level initiations heavily involve the first three chakras, with the focus on clearing issues of safety and survival (first chakra), inner child and sexuality (second chakra), and personal power (third chakra). This then opens you to receive the knowledge that's needed to anchor your consciousness in alignment with Source and puts you in a state of readiness to turn water into wine, heal the multitudes, and ascend. Fairly heady stuff! I teach more about these levels and initiate those who are ready in my 21st Century Energy Medicine Program.

Preparing for Initiation

I still remember the first time I witnessed an initiation. It was my first week apprenticing with a well-known religious teacher, and I was watching him work with a woman in the front of the room. I suddenly felt this incredible wave of energy wash over me and had a strong urge to get down on my knees. I turned to the person sitting next to me and asked what was going on. I was told that it was what they called "slaying in the Spirit" or "bringing down the Holy Spirit." When I saw the very same phenomenon in Mystery School, I was told it was an initiation, or an "awakening of the *kundalini*" (the Sanskrit word for the coiled energy that rests at the base of the spine).

A word of warning: You'll want to be very cautious about the teacher you choose to work with if you believe you may be ready for an initiation. It is possible to force one on someone who isn't ready, and I know of those who do this as a matter of pride. But it is a dangerous practice that can cause the recipient physical, emotional, and spiritual problems. Watch out for any instructor who seems to be operating from ego or is disempowering his or her students. I have seen many individuals get sick while studying with teachers who are coming from ego, so be sure to use your discretion.

❖ ❖

As I previously mentioned, to prepare yourself for an initiation to be stepped up spiritually, you have to do all of that difficult inner work. But what does being ready for one mean? It means that for every curveball that life has thrown at you, you've responded willingly and surrendered to the Divine Plan. Maybe you had a terrible childhood, as I did, or got an illness; or perhaps you had some type of social challenge, such as being overweight, having a stuttering problem, or being extremely shy. It could be that you're really struggling financially or are in the midst of a miserable job or a devastating divorce. Whatever your challenges are, it's how you respond to them that prepares you for an initiation, a spiritual step up.

As the "Serenity Prayer" used by 12-step programs goes: "God grant me the serenity to accept the things I cannot change; courage to change the things I can; and wisdom to know the difference." That's the attitude Spirit is looking for. Not "Why me?" Not being the victim, looking outside yourself to place blame, or getting stuck in bitterness or self-pity.

If you have a regular, effective meditation practice—and I emphasize the word *effective*—that makes it even more likely that you're ready for an upgrade in consciousness. This is one more reason why I always urge people to meditate correctly and every day.

And I'll tell you a little secret about initiations: if one happens to someone in a group you're in, it increases your chances a *thousandfold* of also having one right then and there. That's because once the facilitator brings the higher-level energies into the room, it's easier to move that energy to others who are present and ready. Usually, a few people in the group are what I like to call "low-hanging fruit"—they're totally ripe for an initiation.

What Does an Initiation Do to You?

How do initiations feel? The lower levels, as I've said, can happen without your even realizing it. The higher the initiation level, the more connected you will usually feel, the wilder the experience can be, and the more orgasmic in intensity it is. I'd also like to reiterate that the upper levels are quite physical, and assistance from a facilitator is normally required to achieve them.

Initiation

Each initiation opens and clears the chakras. When you're at the first and second levels, your chakras are cone shaped and open from about 10 to 30 degrees. With each subsequent initiation, those numbers gradually increase, ultimately opening a full 360 degrees. That kind of exposure can cycle the God-force energy optimally. The passageways between the front and back of the chakras are also fully open at that point and become unified, creating a central channel—the vertical power current—that allows energy to move as a vibrational current without any interruption.

Consider how this can affect your life: the more open your chakras are, the better you feel and the more you enjoy life. Really, it's that simple. Plus, this allows you to self-heal more easily. And as for being able to heal others, it's an absolute prerequisite.

While we humans think in linear terms, initiations are from a nonlinear plane. It is possible to be going through more than one at a time, or at least pieces of them, and for them to seem to continue for months, even years, and blend into one another. I've experienced them this way: One time I felt initiatory energy for several years, which made it quite hard to work, as I spent the whole time in a state best described as bliss. Although it was delightful, frankly, it was extremely difficult for me to come back to everyday life when it ended.

Here's a related point: what expands will often later contract. Your energy field and chakras initially expand, but they will later contract, and you will feel smaller, life will look flatter, and it will seem that the guides and gods have all deserted you. If, after the initiation, you could see them and talk to them (and you will be able to as you move up the levels), at one point it will suddenly be as if they have left the planet. This is absolutely the hardest thing to endure. Once you've seen and spoken with Spirit and been intimately linked to it, it's a real downer to have that taken away—it's a truly challenging test, to say the least.

If you've read any biographies of saints from any major religion, you'll find that this experience is shared by every culture. A period of time in the desert—the classic "dark night of the soul," during which you can't seem to connect with anything

149

Divine—often precedes the energy of expansion. So if you feel as if your life couldn't get any worse, and you seem to have been in a dry and barren desert for a long time, you may very well be on the edge of an initiation. And you won't believe the majesty and beauty and connectedness you will feel when you get out of that environment and are initiated.

That's not to say that your problems, the ones you are handling with such grace and acceptance that brought you the initiation in the first place, will go away. If Spirit thinks you need something to keep you humble, your difficulties won't magically disappear. But once you've been initiated, even though you may wake up the next day with the same issues, nothing will look or feel the same ever again. Your concerns will somehow seem smaller. Certainly, you will still feel sadness about a loss or a death, but once you're open and really connected to Source, not much can affect you.

A note about hot flashes: both men and women can get significant hot flashes from an initiatory experience—I certainly did. That's because our bodies are not designed to carry these higher-level vibrations, and it takes some time to adjust to them; otherwise, our energy fields and bodies could burn up.

Keep in mind that some people will be able to have a number of initiations fairly quickly in succession. If you're one of those, you may have a lot of hot flashes—even over a number of years—which will help your body recalibrate to the higher-level vibrations that you're being given. And gals (guys, too!), if you're experiencing hot flashes as a part of aging, don't assume that they are a bad thing; they may, in fact, be a sign that your energy field is recalibrating in anticipation of your next initiation.

If you *do* go through an initiation, be sure to drink lots of water, stay out of the hot sun, and get some extra rest for the next 48 hours afterward. It takes a little while for your field to recalibrate to the higher energies, and these precautions will make the transition a more comfortable one.

Ego and Initiation

Every initiatory level brings with it additional responsibility from that moment on. You are to be even more "in service," and you receive broader power to do your part in this time of world crisis. With increased capability comes the temptation to go into ego, so you're constantly fighting to stay humble as you are given more and more ability. This can be really hard!

One of the biggest hurdles for people who study healing is that they get too attracted to the idea of having initiations, and it becomes a goal. After all, they are the biggest ego boost there is—where, basically, the God-force is saying, "I approve of you." It kind of feels like that moment in the New Testament when the voice came out of the cloud and proclaimed about Jesus: "This is my beloved son, in whom I am well pleased." Really, isn't that the approval we're all secretly craving?

As infants and little children, we project the God source onto our parents—we believe they *are* God. When we're very young, it's easy to remember where we came from because we recently arrived here on Earth, but most of us lose that ability by the time we are five or six years old. For the rest of our lives, we're still looking for that ultimate approval that we tried to get from our parents as stand-ins for God.

When you have an initiation, especially one of the higher ones, it definitely feels like the God force is saying to one and all, "I approve of this person." This can create two problems, the first being that you want the initiation too much. The more you want one, the more unattainable they seem to be. Seriously. So even though I'm giving you this information, your first job will be to learn to "let go and let God," as they say in 12-step programs. Plus, if you want an initiation for the wrong reasons, I guarantee you'll never have one. So if you're seeking one because you're trying to compete—to be "better than"—it simply won't happen.

It's a bit of a catch-22. The more you desire an initiation, the more elusive it becomes. It's similar to wanting a partner: if you seek one out too fervently, to the point of desperation, you scare off any potential mate. The only time I've ever had initiations is when I've completely forgotten all about them and gotten back into fully being of service. And then, *wham!* another one comes out of the blue.

The higher-level initiatory energy seeks out people who serve others, those who "chop wood and carry water," as the Zen proverb says. If you keep putting one foot in front of the other without whining or complaining about your challenges in life, and are always looking for ways to help others, Source will simply seek you out. The best aids for becoming initiation-ready are meditation, prayer, journaling, forgiveness, and being of service. Meditation and prayer put you directly in communication with Source, while journaling puts you in touch with your own emotions and, along with forgiveness, helps you keep clearing out negative energy. And you know already that Spirit has a purpose for those who are dedicated to being of service to others.

The second problem occurs when an individual is ready to move up, takes an initiation, and then loses it. Once lost, it will be much, much harder to regain. My experience is that you're given three tests in the weeks or months following an initiation and, if you fail all three, Source takes it away. I saw this happen to a gifted spiritual teacher who was hands down one of the most clairvoyant people I've ever known. One day he took a big initiation, and afterward found that he could conduct healing energy. Well, his ego grew out of control from having this new power. Before the year was out, he had totally lost not only the healing ability he'd been given, but also his clairvoyance, and he never got either gift back. Talk about humbling!

My most embarrassing initiation/ego story occurred when I'd been working with a shaman for several years as an apprentice. We broke for the summer and, while I was home and going through a particularly difficult time in my life, I had a major initiation with all of the requisite bells and whistles. The day it happened, I saw someone approaching from on high, near the ceiling of the room. At first I thought that perhaps it was a hallucination brought on by the strain I had been going through. When I looked again at the apparition, I suddenly thought, *I recognize that person from somewhere!* Seeing what appeared to be a halo around his head, I then realized it was Jesus. I felt my soul rise from within and say in its own nonverbal language: *I have been waiting for you for such a long time.*

All of the transgressions of my life passed before my eyes in rapid succession, and wave after wave of shame crashed over me as I prayed for forgiveness. As the weight of my petty, self-absorbed, and sordid life was lifted, I understood, as it says in Philippians 4:7, "the peace of God, which surpasses all understanding." An intense rush of ecstasy and joy followed, as all of my senses became heightened and my whole body began to vibrate, which continued for months. It was a beautiful time in my life. I quit working and simply hung out around the ranch. When I would go out in nature, the trees seemed to be waving to me, flowers seemed to smile as I walked by, and I could have sworn the birds were singing a special song just for me. For hours each day, I would sit looking at the view from the cleft of an oak tree on the hillside near my home, simply "being."

During this same period, certain historical figures consistent with my religious upbringing made their presence known. As they worked with me on the inner planes, I learned that I could turn to them for support and direction. In addition to the master healer (Jesus), I spent hours each day in communion with the Madonna and the two Teresas—Saint Teresa of Avila and Saint Thérèse of Lisieux, who is popularly known as "the Little Flower."

After I'd lived in this exalted state for a while, I felt led to sleep outside all night. My husband and I had a mandala (a sacred geometric design) created out of rocks on our ranch property, and I bedded down in the middle of it every evening and kept my gaze on the moon, which I sensed had important lessons for me. After several nights, I became increasingly connected to its energy. One evening in the early fall as I lay under a full harvest moon, I felt an incredible shift in my energy field.

From my training, I knew this passage to be another level of the initiation, and as hard as I tried to resist my urge to feel superior and self-important, I failed. I was secretly sorry that this had occurred during summer vacation—I would have preferred that it happen with the shaman and in front of the other apprentices. After our break, I went back to my training, and my biggest stumbling blocks—competition and pride—found me boasting about my big event to my fellow apprentices. Several days later, the head shaman returned and saw my inflated ego, as if I were wearing a giant sign on my forehead, and promptly sent me to the rear of the healing room and demoted me to work there . . . for a full year! Within moments, I realized my mistake and learned a whole new meaning of the word *humility*. It was very, very humbling.

Thanks to the shaman's quick action, I didn't lose the initiation, even though I *had* failed the first test that Spirit had sent me—to keep my mouth shut about my initiatory experience. I was able to see the subsequent tests coming, and I stayed modest there in the very back of the room.

Then, several years later, all of the signs and wonders stopped. This can often happen before a major initiation—it's another test. My world was once again three-dimensional, and it seemed flat to me. I could not connect with any of my guides, and my intuitive and healing capacities disappeared. I felt abandoned; even worse, I felt like a fraud. Through a desertlike dark night of the soul, I continued my work assisting a prominent healer while I sat humbly in the background, certain that this was to be my only role in this lifetime. I didn't know it in that moment, but this period in the desert was preparing me for the next initiation.

Having the experience of an initiation satisfies the desires of our hearts because, to one degree or another, it connects us to Oneness. It fulfills our deepest longings, the ones we as humans can't quite articulate—to be connected to Source, to God, to All That Is. We come from Source, we are Source, and one day we will all return to Source.

So now that you have learned about initiations, one of the true high points on the journey to becoming your own shaman, we'll conclude by exploring a few of the challenges you may face along the way. The road to becoming your own shaman has its share of obstacles, pitfalls, and difficult questions. Knowing about them ahead of time will help you to see them coming, and allow you to better handle them when they arrive.

chapter ten

WALKING THE PATH

Walking the path of a healer has its ups and downs, as does any path that explores the bright lights and dense shadows of the body and psyche. It takes courage and persistence to be your own shaman. The good news is that you don't have to go it alone. For many of you who want to be healed or heal others, you need flesh-and-blood mentors—teachers who will push you when you need to climb out of the pitfalls of ego; and encourage, comfort, and uplift you when you need support. Beyond that, you have guides on the inner planes who are waiting to assist you—those who will be the beacon that leads you through the dark nights.

Dealing with the Shadow

One of the biggest obstacles we face along the path to shaman-hood is acknowledging and dealing with our shadow side. As I've already explained, we all have one, and some are murkier and denser than others.

Beginning in childhood, we tend to form an idealized self-image that excludes the darker sides of our personality in an attempt to ensure that we will be loved and accepted by others. Unconsciously, we present this partial, "false" self to the world; in the process, we lose touch with important aspects of ourselves that may be less attractive and lovable. However, for our own protection and that of others, when we are working with the powerful energies that are involved in healing, we must learn how to uncover, recognize, and release the shadow aspects of ourselves, as they block our ability to receive and transmit the light that needs to flow through us.

One of the requirements for graduation at the Mystery School I attended involved making a "case presentation," which would offer an opportunity for faculty members to guide students in reclaiming the parts of themselves from which they had split. You see, keeping these aspects of your personality locked away— where you must continually hide, deny, and cover them up, both from yourself and others—requires an enormous amount of energy. In fact, you may spend up to 90 percent of your energy avoiding the things about yourself that you don't want to face. So the intent of the case presentation (which I later learned when I became a teacher was referred to as "walking you to your demise") was for the students to bring about the "death" of their idealized self and become reunited with all of their aspects, and thus, their full power.

I was the first student to step forward in my class. Following the instruction for this section of the final exam, I had chosen a case that had been particularly problematic for me. The point was for me to see what could be learned from my most challenging experience in healing—one where I was off the mark somehow or where things had not turned out well. Because this exercise was important to my graduation as well as my passage into becoming a teacher, and given that I was also quite afraid of public speaking back then, I came to the front of the room with great trepidation to talk about my experience with a man named Roberto. Had I known what was coming—in just a few minutes' time I would experience the demise of my shadow self in front of *a lot* of people— I doubt if I would have had the courage to approach the stage.

Caring for Roberto

I had broken all of the rules about getting too close to Roberto—someone for whom I had played the role of healer. In fact, I had gone so far as to turn my home into a hospice for him.

It had all begun one foggy morning earlier that year. Distraught about being unable to pay his bills, Roberto missed a turn and drove his car off a cliff. He was badly injured, yet he'd managed to crawl back up to the lip of the cliff and was lying in the road. I was on my way to a little chapel not far from my home to meditate in the quiet hours before dawn, driving through the mountains in the darkness, when I saw something that looked like a piece of clothing that had been dropped in the road. As I slowed down to take a closer look, I found a crumpled human being lying there. At once, I slammed on my brakes, jumped out of my car, and ran to his side. A couple also pulled up to help at the same moment and frantically dialed 911 on an early version of a mobile phone. The man on the road was clearly in shock. Having no blanket with me, I cradled his shaking body the best I could with my own body to protect him from the cold.

When I assessed the extent of the man's injuries, I began to panic. His leg was nearly severed just below the knee, and one of his arms lay completely lifeless on the ground. After what seemed like hours (but was probably no more than 30 minutes), the ambulance arrived, and I followed it to the nearest hospital.

While Roberto was recovering, I visited him nearly every day even though the hospital was about an hour away from my house. His arm began to heal, but after four surgeries to save his leg, it was still in fragile condition. On my daily visits to the ICU, I did hands-on healings on my "patient," bobbing and weaving like a total fool in full view of the doctors and nurses. Much to my embarrassment, some of the hospital staff watched with unabashed interest while others politely looked away. But no one ever said a word to me.

One day several months after I'd found that poor man in the road, a hospital administrator phoned me at home. Assuming that

I was his closest relative, he filled me in on Roberto's situation. Being an artist who was visiting the United States from his homeland in the former Czechoslovakia, he had no means of support and no medical insurance, so the hospital had been picking up the tab out of their indigent fund. The man on the phone said that this source was now exhausted, and the hospital would have no choice but to put him out on the street the very next day.

I called to alert my husband—who always quietly tolerates my outrageous behavior—and ran to the rescue. I moved Roberto into the guest room. At this point, he still required twice-daily bandage changes and full-on home care, which I did my best to provide.

As we left the hospital, I bluffed my way through wound-dressing 101, assuring Roberto and the nurse: "I've had plenty of experience changing bandages on horses. I can do this blindfolded," when, in fact, I had dissociated and heard not a word of the nurse's instructions.

Five days later, a home-care nurse came to review the procedure. "Show me what you've been doing," he said.

"Well, I just unwrap the old . . ."

"Wait!" he exclaimed, incredulous. "You have to glove up!"

Horrified to discover that I'd failed to wear protective gloves when changing the bandages, he muttered something about AIDS and hepatitis and urged me to get tested immediately.

After a month of caring for Roberto, I sensed something odd one day during a bandage change. I immediately loaded him into the wheelchair, transferred him to the car, and drove to his surgeon's office. This doctor assured me that all was well, but my intuition knew better. I made a few phone calls and found an infectious-disease specialist in town. I wheeled Roberto into the man's office and insisted that he be seen right away. When the doctor unwrapped the leg, his face turned pale and he looked at me and mouthed, "Gangrene." He immediately admitted Roberto to the hospital, where he stayed for three months, receiving IV antibiotics in a desperate effort to save his leg and his life. With a bit of sleuthing on my part, combined with persuasive tactics from my days as a lawyer, I convinced the hospital administrators to take Roberto back on the basis of a loophole.

My Shadow Side Exposed

The head of the school interrupted my presentation, saying, "You're aware that you broke all of the rules?"

I nodded.

She continued, "We already know that your sense of personal boundaries is impaired given the sexual abuse of your childhood. Can you see how you crossed the line by bringing this stranger into your home and placing his needs above your own and your husband's? Clearly you have a hard time knowing when you're giving too much."

Nodding, I replied, "It's true. I became corded to him the day I found him on the road. We immediately linked energetically."

"A wounded healer like yourself runs a very real risk of becoming improperly bound to another, thus unable to establish realistic limits."

I stood there, nervously trying to maintain my composure and respond with some modicum of personal insight as this woman used her considerable powers from 20 feet away to open me energetically to what I couldn't see. I found myself unable to speak, and an odd sense of vertigo began to come over me. I swallowed hard and blinked my eyes, but my visual field had grown fuzzy around the edges. Suddenly, I saw that Roberto—with all of his foreign, starving-artist charm—had melded with my inner landscape as easily as the blanket of fog had covered the road the morning we'd met.

As I continued with my presentation, still in front of the faculty and members of my class, my mind began to spin. The picture of my life that started to assemble was obviously one I had not been ready or able to see until that very moment. Men like Roberto, who needed my attention more than I did, had lived in my memory as a bunch of odd but disconnected dots. In rapid, quick-cut scenes, all of the males I'd been involved with over the years—boyfriends, lovers, business partners, clients, opposing counsel, and even a judge or two—flashed on the screen of my mind. One by one, I saw their faces and how each dot fit with all the others. Each person had a certain magnetism that had drawn me to him like Little Red Riding Hood was led to a warm, cozy cabin in the woods. Every one of them had an allure, a special debonair flair, a certain darling appeal that could so easily turn needy, much like my father's, and I had never realized this similarity before. They all used their charm to cast a spell over my own approval-seeking side.

Like a cobra rising out of its basket, entranced by the sound of the snake charmer's flute, I was readily controlled and directed by the charisma of men. I did my best to lift them up in my life in whatever way they required; I only needed them to keep up their part of the unspoken bargain and fulfill my need for approval. I reeled as the impact of this pattern began to dawn on me. And then, as if the flute had simply stopped playing, I felt myself begin to fall.

As I lay frozen and helpless on the floor, my own father came front and center in my mental picture, and time seemed to pass in an agonizing fashion as my mind was flooded with childhood memories. I revisited a horrible scene from the summer when I was nine years old, as Daddy's stroking became strangely urgent and I couldn't relieve him in our usual way. He pushed me to the ground, pulled down my pants, and climbed on top of me, muffling my cries with his hand across my mouth. Just as in that terrifying scene, I now lay flat on my back at the front of the room, unable to move as the fear and rage I'd felt toward him, repressed since that day, broke through into consciousness. I began to thrash and scream.

In the midst of this fit, bleary-eyed and red faced, I saw how all of those repressed emotions had led to the formation of my shadow side. In a desperate scramble to survive, I'd become shrewd, manipulative, and at times downright conniving. And yet I'd always thought of myself as merely a harmless control freak.

More of my darkness opened up. The notion that women are the root of all evil was a belief I had all but marinated in while growing up. Between my Portuguese grandmother's view of womankind and my mother's blind eye toward my father's abuse of me, that belief system had seeped into the marrow of my bones: "No matter what a man does, it can always be excused. If he succumbs to his animal instincts, it is surely because the woman led him astray. The man is never at fault, and the woman must guard his awful secrets and jump to fulfill his needs."

As my view of myself as basically good crumbled in the light of the awareness of my own shadow side, I heard the head instructor call for reinforcements—she summoned every guide I knew, plus a few I didn't. With her help, I reconnected with my disowned darkness.

The instructor directed me to harness my displaced energy, which I customarily directed in what is called *the sidewinder pattern*—instead of asking or telling others directly what I wanted from them, I used my personal power in more manipulative ways, such as being deceitful or seductive, to get what I wanted. Before people knew what had hit them, I would get my way. Women will often exhibit strength in this manner, primarily because they fear being crushed by men if they ask for what they want or need candidly. Now, as I lay there on the stage, all of my energy that had been locked down since my childhood was free for me to use, and I was able to move it directly forward through my solar plexus, my power center. I felt like I could move a mountain —two, if necessary —with what was flowing through my body in that moment.

When my awareness returned to the room, the staff and students were standing around me in a half circle as I lay with my arms outstretched in the style of Jesus at the Crucifixion, the archetypal pattern for the fifth initiation. The head teacher looked quite pleased.

Trust Your Instincts; Know Your Boundaries

Another big stumbling block along the path to shamanhood involves your ability to trust yourself and the process, even while undergoing experiences like the one I just described. These events may not be pleasant, yet they could be very necessary for your growth. Becoming your own shaman requires lots of trust, but not blind faith. You have to trust your teachers while not giving away your power to them. You must trust that the trail you're on will lead you to the mountaintop, yet you will have to slog through many a valley to get there.

The path of the healer is not clear-cut; there are no memos to tell you what to do and no course laid out in stone to follow. There are simply hints and glimmers of what lies ahead, whispers in the night, a voice in the wind as it calls your name. So what you have to trust the most is *you*. You need to have faith that you really are in contact with your invisible guides, even when you can't see or hear them. You must be confident that what you see or feel in another person is really what needs to be healed, and then possess the belief in your ability to effect change on all levels of his or her being. You also have to give credence to the subtle messages that you receive about your own life.

Yet it is equally important not to relinquish your skepticism and your rational mind. You still need to pay the rent or mortgage; take care of your body; and function in your role as parent, partner, or worker. You have to learn how to maintain boundaries so that you are not taking on the issues of others or expecting others to take care of yours. You must filter the messages you receive from beyond this plane to know whether they are indeed meant for your highest good.

In order to give up a lucrative law career so that I could go chasing sages and shamans around the world and learn from them, I had to have a compelling belief that I wasn't crazy. I had to forget about what I looked like, what others thought about me. For example, I remember the year I received subtle signals to practice sounding, which I talked about in some detail in Chapter 8. I would stand outside and gaze at the horizon as I made vocalizations for hours at a time, my voice changing from low to high, over and over again, and I was fortunate to not have neighbors close by. Not long afterward, as you know, I started using this technique as a way to initiate others into elevated levels of spirituality.

So how do you learn to trust yourself, to rely on those messages you receive? You build confidence in your connection to Source based on past experience. Maybe you listened to your inner voice when it told you that it was time to move to another state—even though you loved where you were living—and it turned out to be a really good move. Or maybe you chose not to hear the inner prompting that said: *Stay away from that person,* and you realized later that you should have honored that feeling in your gut. Or perhaps you felt that you were visited by your grandmother who passed over many years ago, which was confirmed by someone who could see her clairvoyantly.

Eventually, through such validations, you learn to rely on your inner promptings, especially when they come to you while you're in a clear space—immediately after meditation, for example. Some people learn to trust the messages they receive in vivid dreams, while others pay attention to instincts. Whatever your channel of communication with Source, your life will be more purposeful and meaningful, richer and fuller, when you come to trust yourself.

Healing vs. Curing

One of the most important questions you will deal with in your quest to walk the path of the shaman has to do with who gets healed versus who gets cured. And it's not an easy one, as it can derail your faith in yourself.

While wandering through the woods in the winter of 1858, a shepherd girl named Marie-Bernarde Soubirous saw a beautiful lady in a flowing white robe near a small grotto along the banks of the river Gave de Pau in France. The daughter of devout Christian peasants, the 14-year-old known as Bernadette eventually saw the lady a total of 18 times. The woman told the young girl to advise her village priest to construct a chapel on the site of the encounter. On March 25, 1858, on the occasion of the 16th visitation, the lady revealed herself to be none other than the Blessed Virgin. In an ecstatic trance, Bernadette rose from her knees, walked a few steps, and fell back to the earth, where she began to scrape the ground until a small rivulet of water formed a puddle in the dirt. In the days that followed, the puddle formed a sacred spring and pool that is now the famous healing shrine at Lourdes.

Although Mary told Bernadette that the waters would heal people, the spring did not cure this sickly girl, who suffered from debilitating asthma until her death at an early age. And yet, for 30 years after she passed, Bernadette's corpse did not decay. To this day, Lourdes is the most visited shrine in all of Christendom, with some six million people making the pilgrimage each year. Within the first 50 years, roughly 4,000 miracle healings were recorded.

Of the 10,000 people who visit the spring at Lourdes each day, why do some dance away from the sacred waters while others depart still dependent on crutches? Why is one woman relieved of alcoholism, never to drink again, while another person who also attends her 12-step group religiously and stays sober for many years suddenly falls off the wagon, stays drunk, and ultimately dies of liver failure? Why do some people get the message, grace, miraculous reprieve, or spontaneous remission . . . and others do not?

As shamans and healers, we make a distinction between a *cure*—physical recovery and elimination of a disease condition— and a *healing,* which can occur on spiritual and emotional levels and may not involve a correlating physical resolution. Ideally, both will take place.

The Mystery School I attended taught that the higher self or soul of an individual ultimately makes the choice as to whether or not someone will physically heal. To an extent, I believe this is true. However, I saw that students often took the low road when a physical cure didn't manifest. Many of them would step back and accept too readily that a tangible result had not occurred, rather than work diligently on raising their own vibratory ability to bring more juice—a stronger connection to Source with a higher potential for healing—to their work. The explanation provided in that environment was: "Your client's higher self knows best and will decide whether or not to be cured. You, the healer, are not responsible for the choice of the client's soul."

I have given this a great deal of thought over the years, and I am bothered when the explanation serves as an easy way out for the healer when a cure doesn't take place. For a period of time, it was convenient for me to excuse my own failures to effect a cure based on the idea that the client had decided at a soul level not to accept the help. But some part of me remained unconvinced, and I continued to grapple with the issue.

What I've come to believe, after working on many tens of thousands of people, is that it is uncommon for someone who is seeking to be cured of a physical condition to be at the point where his or her soul has said, "Time's up—I need to leave." So I've swung back to my original training: I believe that it's the healer's job to make it happen. In my early apprenticeship with Christian healers, I was deeply impressed by the work of Agnes Sanford. In her book *The Healing Light,* she explains: "Let us understand then that if our [healing] experiment fails, it is not due to a lack in God, but to a natural and understandable lack in ourselves." This puts responsibility squarely on the shoulders of the healer.

Suppose I decide to try firewalking and several people in front of me make it across the burning surface without so much as a blister, but my attempt forces me to jump off the red-hot coals with third-degree burns. Are the coals at fault? Self-responsibility requires that I look at my state of mind and heart at the moment I took my first step.

Invariably, in the world of healing there are many individuals who are not physically cured even though they might be emotionally and spiritually healed, and I am constantly humbled by these failures. Fortunately, thanks to those who have successfully walked across the coals ahead of me—Mary Baker Eddy, Agnes Sanford, and Kathyrn Kuhlman, for example—I'm reminded that miraculous healings are indeed possible. This brings me back again and again to focus on my responsibility to forge a stronger and more reliable connection with Divine power.

The Mountaintop

Whether we're looking to heal ourselves or acquire the ability to heal others, the path of the shaman always leads to the same goal: connecting to, and eventually merging with, Oneness—the summit of all our yearnings and desires. One taste of Source is usually enough to put our feet on the path for the rest of our lives and take one step after another as we climb the foothills and traverse the valleys that will one day take us to our true home.

As difficult as the journey may be, one upon which you'll experience both tears of pain and tears of joy, there is nothing on Earth that can compare to it. You will understand that your life has a noble and honorable purpose. You will know that what you do helps to relieve the suffering of humanity as well as yourself. You will be in alignment with Divine Will and the Divine Plan. You will have a much broader and more compassionate view of all of life. And you will feel free—a deep and gratifying freedom—no matter what your actual circumstances might look like to anyone else.

I will look for you along the road. . . .

EPILOGUE

When looking down from the spiritual plane, you decide to reincarnate and then work in consultation with your guides to choose your parents, your work, and the issues you want to address this time around. Initially, you bring only a small portion of your total consciousness to inhabit your physical body. The rest of it, your higher self, remains outside of the body. In this lifetime, you are separated from it and the qualities it contains unless you embark on initiations that allow you to access more of this part of your being—your God Self.

Your entire body was designed to help you transform your consciousness in order to do just that. Every system of your body—from the endocrine to the cardiovascular to the nervous—is specially designed to assist you in progressing spiritually. Using your physical aspects and your energy field, you continue to work at that purpose throughout your life, hopefully striving to reach beyond your small self and access more and more of your expanded awareness with each challenging situation you encounter. If you're successful, you'll move to higher and higher energetic levels. But if you throw in the towel and give up when the going gets tough, becoming whiny or resentful or full of self-pity while blaming others for your problems, chances are that after death you'll find yourself stuck in a world that feels just like the worst days you had here. Some call this *hell*.

However, each time you bring in more of "you," more of your higher self from the chakras that are above your head, you fulfill your soul's desire to be transformed. That yearning to incorporate more of your finest qualities is part of your soul's deep longing to reconnect with the God-force from which it came and of which it is a part.

You are in the process of clearing yourself and becoming more of God every moment of every day. As you continue to move up spiritually, your energies will be focused less and less on the petty and the negative, and more and more on love.

My love is healing. Perhaps yours will be, too!

APPENDIX

21st Century Energy Medicine Program

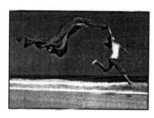 Embark on a journey into the mysterious world of energy medicine. In this premier program, you will learn healing techniques, advanced divination skills, how to connect to your spirit guides, and how to meditate effectively. Come participate in the ancient rites and secrets of the shamanic realm, as this program leads you in awakening your inner healer.

If you're looking for a new professional opportunity, this program also offers a certification in Energy Medicine that can launch your career as an energy healer.

For complete details, please visit: **www.deborahkingcenter** **.com/energy** or call 800-790-5785 for more information.

The Shamanic Pendulum Kit

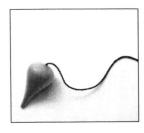

Read the invisible with this Shamanic Pendulum Kit that has everything you need to become an expert dowser. Handmade and blessed by humble craftsmen and personally selected by Deborah King, this kit includes instructions and a chakra chart that will guide you in its use. It's perfect for both divining your future and interpreting the movement of the chakras.

To order this pendulum kit, please visit: **www.deborahking center.com/ShamanicPendulumKit** or call 800-790-5785.

INDEX

Index

❖ ❖ ❖ ❖

ACKNOWLEDGMENTS

This project could not have been accomplished without the support, guidance, and influence of many people. Much gratitude goes to the following key individuals:

My editors—Jill Kramer, Shannon Littrell, and Patrick Gabrysiak—and everyone at Hay House . . . they're the best!

Brookes Nohlgren and Parvati Markus, for their unflagging editing skills, helping me turn my chapters into one cohesive whole.

Scott Hartley, fellow teacher, marketing expert, tech genius, musician, and friend who's always there for me—he gets a big thank-you.

Marilyn Warren, longtime friend, for keeping the office running smoothly 24/7 and for being so supportive.

Chris Raj, for his tech support and help in the field.

Jan Stake, for her accounting expertise and friendship.

Terri Jay, for her patient listening and enduring friendship.

Carl Studna, photographer extraordinaire, thank you for my photo.

But most of all, this book and my work would not be possible without my husband, Eric, who is always by my side.

ABOUT THE AUTHOR

Master healer and teacher **Deborah King** was a successful attorney in her 20s when a diagnosis of cancer sent her on a search for truth that radically changed her life. Unwilling to undergo invasive surgery, she turned to alternative medicine and had an amazing remission at the hands of a healer. Along the way, she conquered the alcohol and drug addictions she had used to bury an abusive childhood. Leaving the corporate arena for the mysterious world of healers, sages, and shamans, Deborah mastered ancient and modern healing systems, ultimately developing a powerful healing technique of her own.

Combining her personal history and wisdom, Deborah wrote the national bestseller *Truth Heals: What You Hide Can Hurt You,* which explores the powerful relationship between the suppression of painful emotions and their impact on our health and happiness.

Deborah travels worldwide, helping thousands of people transform their lives through her experiential workshops. Her online training course, the 21st Century Energy Medicine Program, attracts those who want to become adept healers for themselves and others. She also hosts a popular weekly Hay House Radio show.

Website: **www.deborahkingcenter.com**

NOTES

NOTES

We hope you enjoyed this Hay House book. If you'd like
to receive our online catalog featuring additional information
on Hay House books and products, or if you'd like to find
out more about the Hay Foundation, please contact:

Hay House, Inc., P.O. Box 5100, Carlsbad, CA 92018-5100
(760) 431-7695 or (800) 654-5126
(760) 431-6948 (fax) or (800) 650-5115 (fax)
www.hayhouse.com® • **www.hayfoundation.org**

❖ ❖

Published and distributed in Australia by: Hay House Australia
Pty. Ltd., 18/36 Ralph St., Alexandria NSW 2015 • *Phone:* 612-9669-4299
Fax: 612-9669-4144 • www.hayhouse.com.au

Published and distributed in the United Kingdom by: Hay House UK,
Ltd., 292B Kensal Rd., London W10 5BE • *Phone:* 44-20-8962-1230
Fax: 44-20-8962-1239 • www.hayhouse.co.uk

Published and distributed in the Republic of South Africa by:
Hay House SA (Pty), Ltd., P.O. Box 990, Witkoppen 2068
Phone/Fax: 27-11-467-8904 • www.hayhouse.co.za

Published in India by: Hay House Publishers India, Muskaan Complex,
Plot No. 3, B-2, Vasant Kunj, New Delhi 110 070 • *Phone:* 91-11-4176-1620
Fax: 91-11-4176-1630 • www.hayhouse.co.in

Distributed in Canada by: Raincoast, 9050 Shaughnessy St.,
Vancouver, B.C. V6P 6E5 • *Phone:* (604) 323-7100
Fax: (604) 323-2600 • www.raincoast.com

❖ ❖

<u>Take Your Soul on a Vacation</u>

Visit **www.HealYourLife.com**® to regroup, recharge,
and reconnect with your own magnificence.
Featuring blogs, mind-body-spirit news, and
life-changing wisdom from Louise Hay and friends.

Visit **www.HealYourLife.com** today!

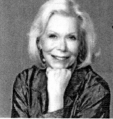
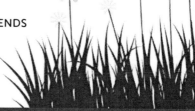

CPSIA information can be obtained at www.ICGtesting.com
Printed in the USA
BVOW04s1231110516

447648BV00001B/35/P